Psychiatry pocket

G000165522

1
2
3

Author:
S. K. Shivakumar MD, MRCPsych (UK), FRCPC(C)
Assistant Professor Department of Psychiatry
Northern Ontario School of Medicine Sudbury Regional Hospital
680 Kirkwood Drive
Sudbury P3E 2X2
Canada

Acknowledgements:

Dr. Kathleen Anderson   Dr. Angela Gola   Dr. Angelita Sanchez
Dr. Ranga Shivakumar   Dr. Kuldip Jassal   Dr. Rayudu Koka
Dr. Shabir Amanullah

Editing: Sharyu Gangwal, MD, Dominik Stauber, MD, Jayateerth Korti, MD, Daniel Nichita, MD
Cover Illustration: Saket Sisodia, Alexander Storck, Petra Rau, Trupti Pawnikar
Production: Alexander Storck, Petra Rau
Publisher: Börm Bruckmeier Publishing LLC, www.media4u.com

Printed in China by Colorcraft Ltd., Hong Kong
ISBN 978-1-59103-262-5

Preface

The art of learning psychiatry is constantly evolving. Covering the whole breadth of psychiatry, this concise, yet comprehensive **Psychiatry pocket** guide serves to bring the readers up-to-date knowledge required to deal with patients with psychiatric illnesses. It is an easy to use guide with logically structured chapters containing the latest advances and guidelines in psychiatry. This pocket guide is an essential quick reference for psychiatric clerks, residents, fellows in training, as well as experienced practicing psychiatrist and health professionals who come into contact with psychiatric patients.

The **Psychiatry pocket** is divided into 13 chapters, guiding the readers in an easy to follow style, offering evidenced based guidance on management and treatment issues. Each of the chapters provides adequate coverage of most commonly seen psychiatric disorders in day to day clinical practice. Topics covered range from the most commonly seen psychiatric disorders including anxiety, mood disorders, and schizophrenia to psychopharmacology.

For easy and quick access, the **Psychiatry pocket** includes treatment guidelines, algorithms and several handy tables detailing the commonly used psychiatric medications as well as other information that need not be committed to memory.

We hope that you will find the book helpful in providing comprehensive quality care for patients with psychiatric disorders.

We welcome critical comments and constructive suggestions from the readers. Please contact us at info@media4u.com

We would like to acknowledge the following people for their contributions to this book:

Dr. Kathleen Anderson   Dr. Angela Golas   Dr. Angelita Sanchez
Dr. Ranga Shivakumar   Dr. Kuldip Jassal   Dr. Rayudu Koka
Dr. Shabir Amanullah

The author and publisher   September, 2012

S. K. Shivakumar, MD

Contents

Contents

Contents

1   General Principles

1.1   The Psychiatric Evaluation

1.1.1   Psychiatric History

Psychiatric History	
Identifying Data	Name, age, sex, language, marital status, living status, occupation
Chief Complaint (CC)	Reason why patient has come for help, in the patient's own words
History of Present Illness (HPI)	Narrative description of the course and chronology of symptoms: onset, symptoms, changes at home or at work, setting, problems with family or friends
Past Psychiatric History	Past episodes that have required psychiatric care (presenting symptoms, extent of incapacity, type of treatment, names of doctors and hospitals involved)
Past Medical History (PMH)	Past medical problems/operations, current medical problems, allergies, current medications
Substance Abuse	Current or past use of alcohol, nicotine, opiates, amphetamines, benzodiazepines (test CAGE = Cutting down, Annoyed, Guilty, Eye opener)
Family and Marital History	Marital status, children, relationship with the patient, other family members with psychiatric/medical problems
Social History	Living situation, education, occupation, income, encounters with the law

1.1.2   Psychopathology Evaluation

Psychopathology Assessment	
Consciousness	Reduced, clouded, narrowed, expanded
Orientation	Time, place, situation, self
Attention, Memory	Apperception, concentration ("100−7=..."), memorization (apple-table-cello), retention, confabulations, paramnesias; impaired memorization and ocular motor function: consider Wernicke´s encephalopathy!

Psychopathology Assessment (cont.)	
Formal Thought Disorders	• **Thinking**: Inhibited, retarded, circumstantial, restricted; • **Formal order**: Perseveration, rumination, pressured thinking, flight of ideas, tangential thinking, blocking, incoherence; • **Perception and abstract thinking**: Explain proverbs; neologisms
Phobias and Compulsions	Suspiciousness, hypochondriasis (non-delusional), phobias, obsessive thoughts, compulsive impulses, compulsive actions
Delusions	**Ask specific questions!** • **Often in schizophrenia**: Delusions of reference, persecution • **Often in affective psychosis**: Delusions of guilt or of poverty, hypochondriacal delusions • **Often in manic DO or schizophrenia**: Delusions of grandeur • **Additional delusions**: Delusional mood, (sudden) delusional ideas, systemic delusions, delusional dynamics, delusional jealousy, other delusions
Perception	Illusions; hallucinations: Verbal, auditory, visual, bodily, olfactory
Loss of Ego Boundaries	Derealization, depersonalization, thought broadcasting, withdrawal, thought insertion, other symptoms
Disturbances of Affect	• **Depressive disorder**: Perplexity, loss of feeling, blunted affect, depressed mood, hopelessness, anxiety, inadequacy, feelings of guilt, feelings of impoverishment • **Manic disorder**: Euphoria, dysphoria, irritability, exaggerated self-esteem • **Schizophrenia**: Ambivalence, parathymia • **Organic disorder**: Affective lability/ incontinence; • **Other disorder**: Loss of vitality, restlessness, complaintive, affective rigidity
Psychomotor Disturbances	• **Volition**: Lack of drive, inhibition • **Motor activity:** Motor restlessness, parakinesia, mannerisms, histrionic • **Speech:** Mutism, logorrhea **Catatonic symptoms:** Negativism, stupor, waxy flexibility
Introspection? Insight? Suicidal thoughts: Ask specific questions!	
Other Disturbances	
Social	Social withdrawal, excessive social contact, aggressiveness
Other	Suicidal tendencies, self-mutilation, no sense of feeling ill, lack of insight, uncooperative, lack of self-care

Somatic Symptoms	
Sleep/Vigilance	Difficulties falling asleep, interrupted sleep, shortened sleep, waking early, drowsiness, circadian disturbances (often in depressive disorders)
Appetite	Decreased or excessive appetite, excessive thirst, decreased libido
Gastrointestinal	Hypersalivation, dry mouth, nausea, vomiting, gastric discomfort, constipation, diarrhea
Cardiopulmonary	Breathing difficulties, dizziness, palpitations, cardiac pain
Autonomic	Increased perspiration, seborrhea, urination difficulties, menstrual difficulties
Σ : Summarize all symptoms > multiaxial diagnosis	

1.2   Multiaxial Assessment

1.2.1   Introduction

The complex interplay of medical, emotional, social and cultural factors in the genesis of psychiatric disease requires the clinician to conduct a careful examination of many different facets of the patient's life and function. It is important to consider not only medical causes, but also the patient's overall performance socially, occupationally, academically, in family life, as well as maladaptive behavior such as substance abuse, impaired coping skills, and so on.

This broad approach to the examination of an individual is most appropriately undertaken using **a multiaxial assessment** whereby different components of the patient's mental and functional condition are evaluated in different categories, or axes. Use of a multiaxial system facilitates comprehensive and systematic evaluation of functioning capacity, potential mental and medical disorders, and psychosocial and environmental problems, items that might otherwise be overlooked if the focus was solely on assessing the primary presenting problem.

The Diagnostic Statistical Manual (DSM) uses a 5-axis multiaxial classification as its framework in the evaluation of the psychiatric patient. This approach is described in more detail in the sections that follow.

Other multiaxial frameworks are also available. For example, The Standardized Multiaxial Formulation of the World Psychiatric Association (WPA), uses a 4-axis approach to achieve a similar objective.

1.2.2 The DSM Multiaxial Classification

DSM–IV Multiaxial Classification	
Axis I	• Clinical psychiatric disorders • Other conditions that may be a focus of clinical attention
Axis II	• Personality disorders • Mental retardation
Axis III	General medical conditions
Axis IV	Psychosocial and environmental problems
Axis V	Global assessment of functioning

1.2.3 DSM Axis I – Clinical Disorders

Axis I – Clinical Disorders

Axis I is for recording the primary clinical disorder or disorders. Essentially, every psychiatric diagnosis, with the exception of personality disorders and mental retardation which are coded on Axis II, is recorded here. Multiple Axis I disorders may be diagnosed, but the primary diagnosis should be listed first. General categories are listed below:

- Disorders usually first diagnosed in infancy, childhood, or adolescence (excluding mental retardation, which is diagnosed on Axis II)
- Delirium, dementia, amnesia and other cognitive disorders
- Mental disorders due to a general medical condition
- Substance-related disorders
- Schizophrenia and other psychotic disorders
- Mood disorders
- Anxiety disorders
- Somatoform disorders
- Factitious disorders
- Dissociative disorders
- Sexual and gender identity disorders
- Eating disorders
- Sleep disorders
- Impulse-control disorders
- Adjustment disorders
- Other conditions that may be a focus of clinical attention

1.2.4   DSM Axis II – Personality Disorders and Mental Retardation

Axis II – Personality Disorders and Mental Retardation

Used to report personality disorders and mental retardation. Axis II may also be used for noting prominent maladaptive personality features and defense mechanisms. Multiple disorders may be reported. General disorder categories to be reported here are listed below:

- Paranoid personality disorder
- Narcissistic personality disorder
- Schizoid personality disorder
- Avoidant personality disorder
- Schizotypal personality disorder
- Dependent personality disorder
- Antisocial personality disorder
- Obsessive-compulsive personality disorder
- Borderline personality disorder
- Histrionic personality disorder
- personality disorder NOS
- Mental retardation

1.2.5   DSM Axis III – General Medical Conditions

Axis III – General Medical Conditions

- Used to report general medical conditions that are directly or indirectly related to the mental disorder, or that may potentially be relevant to understanding or managing the person's mental disorder. For example, hypothyroidism may directly cause depression, whereas a diagnosis of breast carcinoma may indirectly cause depression.
- In cases where the mental disorder is directly and clearly caused by a medical condition, the condition may also be recorded on Axis I as Mental Disorder due to a General Medical Condition, with the condition specified. In cases where the link is unclear or indirect, the condition should only be recorded on Axis III.

1.2.6   DSM Axis IV– Psychosocial and Environmental Problems

Axis IV – Psychosocial and Environmental Problems

Axis IV is for reporting psychosocial and environmental problems that may affect the diagnosis, treatment, and prognosis of mental disorders. Typically, these are stressful negative events (such as depression caused by death of a loved one or job loss), but occasionally they can be positive events (such as a panic disorder triggered after admission to medical school). These may occasionally be coded on Axis I under Other Conditions That May be a Focus of Clinical Attention, if they are the primary problem. Typical psychosocial problems are included below:

| Primary support group | Death of loved one, divorce, estrangement, health problems in family, sexual or physical abuse, neglect, discipline issues, sibling birth or discord |

Axis IV - Psychosocial and Environmental Problems (cont.)	
Social environment	Inadequate social support, living alone, life-cycle transition problems (eg, retirement), acculturation problems, discrimination, death of a friend
Educational	Illiteracy, academic difficulties, discord with teachers or classmates, inadequate educational environment
Occupational	Unemployment, threat of job loss, job and career dissatisfaction, difficult work conditions, supervisor or coworker discord, changing jobs
Housing	Homelessness, inadequate housing, overcrowded housing, lack of privacy, unsafe neighborhood, discord with neighbors or landlord
Economic	Extreme poverty, inadequate finances, insufficient welfare support
Access to health care services	Inadequate health care services, unavailable transportation to health care facilities, inadequate health insurance
Crime and legal system	Arrest, incarceration, litigation, victim of crime
Miscellaneous	Exposure to traumatic event, disasters, war, other hostilities, discord with nonfamily caregivers such as counselor, social worker, or physician, unavailability of social service agencies

1.2.7   DSM Axis V – Global Assessment of Functioning

Axis V - Global Assessment of Functioning
Axis V is for reporting the clinician's judgment of the individual's overall level of functioning. This information is useful in planning treatment, measuring its impact, and predicting outcome. The level of functioning may be measured using the GAF Scale.

The Global Assessment of Functioning (GAF) Scale

- Use only to rate global psychological, social, and occupational functioning. **Do not include impairment in functioning due to physical or environmental limitations.**
- Assign GAF score in the range that best matches the individual's symptoms **OR** level of functioning, **whichever is worse.**
- The evaluation should consider a recent finite interval, such as the previous week or month. Indicate in parenthesis after the score the time period the score reflects, eg, "(current)", "(at discharge)", "(highest level in past month)".

The Global Assessment of Functioning (GAF) Scale (cont.)	
Score	Description of Symptoms and Global Functioning
91–100	No symptoms. Superior functioning in a wide range of activities, life's problems never seem to get out of hand, is sought out by others because of his or her many positive qualities.
81–90	Absent or minimal symptoms (eg, mild anxiety before an exam), good functioning in all areas, interested and involved in a wide range of activities, socially effective, generally satisfied with life, no more than everyday problems or concerns (eg, an occasional argument with family members).
71–80	If symptoms are present, they are transient and expectable reactions to psychosocial stressors (eg, difficulty concentrating after family argument), no more than slight impairment in social, occupational, or school functioning (eg, temporarily falling behind in schoolwork).
61–70	Some mild symptoms (eg, depressed mood and mild insomnia) OR some difficulty in social, occupational, or school functioning (eg, occasional truancy, or theft within the household), but generally functioning pretty well, has some meaningful interpersonal relationships.
51–60	Moderate symptoms (eg, flat affect and circumstantial speech, occasional panic attacks) OR moderate difficulty in social, occupational, or school functioning (eg, few friends, conflicts with peers or coworkers).
41–50	Serious symptoms (eg, suicidal ideation, severe obsessional rituals, frequent shoplifting) OR any serious impairment in social, occupational, or school functioning (eg, no friends, unable to keep a job).
31–40	Some impairment in reality testing or communication (eg, speech is at times illogical, obscure, or irrelevant) OR major impairment in several areas, such as work or school, family relations, judgment, thinking, or mood (eg, depressed man avoids friends, neglects family, and is unable to work; child frequently beats up younger children, is defiant at home, and is failing at school).
21–30	Behavior is considerably influenced by delusions or hallucinations OR serious impairment in communication or judgment (eg, sometimes incoherent, acts grossly inappropriately, suicidal preoccupation) OR inability to function in almost all areas (eg, stays in bed all day; no job, home, or friends).

The Global Assessment of Functioning (GAF) Scale (cont.)	
Score	Description of Symptoms and Global Functioning
11–20	Some danger of hurting self or others (eg, suicide attempts without clear expectation of death; frequently violent; manic excitement) OR occasionally fails to maintain minimal personal hygiene (eg, smears feces) OR gross impairment in communication (eg, largely incoherent or mute).
1–10	Persistent danger of severely hurting self or others (eg, recurrent violence) OR persistent inability to maintain minimal personal hygiene OR serious suicidal act with clear expectation of death.
0	Inadequate information.

Endicott J, Spitzer RL, Fleiss JL, Cohen J. The Global Assessment Scale: A Procedure for Measuring Overall Severity of Psychiatric Disturbance. Archives of General Psychiatry 33:766–771, 1976). A modified version of the GAS was included in DSM-ILL-R as the Global Assessment of Functioning (GAF) Scale.

1.2.8   WPA Standardized Multiaxial Formulation

Another multiaxial approach is the Standardized Multiaxial Formulation devised by the World Psychiatric Association (WPA) International Guidelines for Diagnostic Assessment (IGDA) Working Group. Similarly to the multiaxial approach used in the DSM, this framework examines various areas of the individual's medical and mental health, functioning in various areas of life, disability profile, and general quality of life. As with the DSM, the objective is to use a thorough and systematic assessment to obtain a comprehensive picture of the patient's condition.

Standardized Multiaxial Formulation (WPA-IGDA)	
Axis I – Clinical Disorders	
A. Mental disorders	Record the **ICD-10 codes** for each mental or medical disorder the patient presents with.
B. General medical disorders	
Axis II – Disabilities in Functioning	
A. Personal care and survival	• **Score** severity of disability in each category on a scale **from 0 to 5** (mild to massive)*
B. Occupational functioning	• The **WHO Disability Diagnostic Scale** may also be used →19
C. Family functioning	
D. Broad social functioning	• Add the scores for each category to obtain a total disability score

Standardized Multiaxial Formulation (WPA-IGDA)	
Axis III - Contextual Psychosocial Problems	
1. Family/housing	For each of these categories, enter the **ICD-10 Z-codes** for any psychosocial problems pertinent to the presentation, course or treatment of the patient's disorders or relevant to clinical care, as well as personal problems such as hazardous, violent, abusive and suicidal behaviors that do not fall under a standard disorder.
2. Educational/work	
3. Economic/legal	
4. Cultural/environmental	
5. Personal	
Axis IV - Quality of Life	
• Score from 0 to 10 the quality of life perceived by the patient: **0 = Poor and 10 = Excellent** • The score may be determined by an appropriate multidimensional instrument or by direct global rating	

*Disability scoring: 0-none; 1-medium; 2-moderate; 3-substantial; 4-severe; 5-massive; U-unknown

1.2.9 The WHO Disability Diagnostic Scale

WHO Disability Diagnostic Scale (WHO-DDS)
Instructions
• Each functioning area should be scored using the scoring system indicated below using the best estimate of the degree of dysfunction in relation to the maximum level of expected functioning in the sociocultural context of the patient. • The rating should be made regardless of whether the dysfunction is due to somatic or psychiatric conditions, but the main reason for dysfunction should also be indicated (mainly psychiatric, mainly somatic, both somatic and psychiatric). • The functional disability scores should be recorded on **Axis II of the WPA Standardized Multiaxial Formulation.**

Functional Areas	
A	Personal care and survival
B	Occupational functioning: Performance of expected role as remunerated worker, student or homemaker
C	Functioning with family: Interaction with spouse, parents, children and other relatives
D	Broader social behavior (functioning in other roles and activities): Interaction with other individuals and the community-at-large, leisure activities

WHO Disability Diagnostic Scale (WHO–DDS) (cont.)

Score	Definitions
0	No dysfunction: The patient's functioning conforms to the norms of his/her reference group or sociocultural context.
20	Minimum dysfunction: Deviation from the norm in one or more activities/roles is present. The disturbances are minor but persist over the greater part of the time period. More conspicuous dysfunctions may appear for very short periods, eg, one or two days.
40	Obvious dysfunction: The deviation from the norm is conspicuous and dysfunctions interfere with social adjustment. Dysfunction in at least one activity/role persists nearly all the time. More severe dysfunction may appear only for a few days.
60	Serious dysfunction: Deviations from the norm are marked in most activities/roles and persist more than half of the time.
80	Very serious dysfunction: Deviation in all areas are very severe and persist nearly all the time. Action by others to remedy or control the dysfunction might be required (according to the rater's judgment), but it does not need to have taken place in order to make this rating.
99	Maximum dysfunction: Deviation from the norm has reached a crisis point. A clear element of danger to the patient's own existence or social life and/or to the lives of others may be present. Some form of action or social intervention is necessary.
XX	Not applicable (state reason)

1.3 Classification and Diagnostic Systems

There are two major diagnostic classification systems in psychiatry, the **International Classification of Disease, 10th revision (ICD-10)** and the **Diagnostic Statistical Manual, 4th edition, Text Revision (DSM-IV-TR).**

The ICD is a global disease classification system created over a century ago and maintained by the World Health Organization (WHO). The latest revision, the ICD-10, was completed in 1992 and is in wide use throughout the world. It contains diagnostic classification for every medical condition, with mental and behavioral conditions being addressed in Chapter V. The next revision, the ICD-11, is currently being drafted and is scheduled for publication in 2015.

The DSM-IV-TR is published by the American Psychiatric Association (APA) and addresses only mental and behavioral disorders and related conditions. The DSM was first published in 1952, and has undergone several revisions with the latest, the DSM-IV-TR, being published in 2000. The DSM-IV-TR is currently the primary psychiatric diagnostic manual used in the United States. The next revision of the DSM, the DSM-V, is anticipated in 2013.

The United States is scheduled to transition from ICD-9 to ICD-10 starting in October of 2013 as of this writing. A modified version of the ICD-10, referred to as the ICD-10 Clinical Modification, or ICD-10-CM, will be used in the US. While the ICD will not immediately replace the DSM in US mental health, it is nonetheless important for health professionals to be familiar with the ICD-10 mental disorder coding system and diagnostic criteria.

This book uses both the ICD-10 and DSM-IV-TR classification and diagnostic systems, whenever possible. We hope that the book will serve as a bridge between these two systems, and that this dual use will be a useful resource in the diagnosis and management of psychiatric disease.

2 Psychosis and Schizophrenia

2.1 Psychotic Symptoms

Psychosis is a disturbance in the perception of reality that can manifest with hallucinations, delusions or thought disorganization. Other symptoms include agitation, impulsivity, aggression, loss of ego boundaries, and other forms of behavioral dysfunction. Severe psychosis renders the patient nonfunctional, poses a significant danger to self and others, and requires immediate hospitalization and treatment.

2.1.1 Hallucinations

Hallucinations are **false sensory perceptions** in the absence of external stimuli and may be auditory, visual or other sensory (eg, tactile, olfactory).

- Auditory hallucinations are the most common type of hallucinations in schizophrenia (present in 40%-80% of patients). Such hallucinations are perceived as voices or sounds in the absence of an external source, and are distinct from the person's own thoughts. They have often been described as a cacophony or chorus of voices that are either not intelligible, or if they are, are of a persecutory or derogatory nature
- Hallucinations can also involve other senses including visual hallucinations (usually indistinct patterns or colors, but occasionally distinct forms, faces, or people), somatic hallucinations (the feeling of being touched), and more rarely, olfactory hallucinations
- Hallucinations are a prominent feature of the paranoid type of schizophrenia

2.1.2 Delusions

Delusions are **false beliefs** that are firmly held despite obvious evidence to the contrary, and are not typical of the patient's culture, faith, or family. Various methods for classifying delusions include the following:

Classification of Delusions	
Bizarre vs non bizarre	
Bizarre	Bizarre delusions are clearly implausible (eg, aliens are communicating with the patient through the television)
Non bizarre	Plausible but unlikely delusions such as various persecutorial or paranoid delusions (eg, extreme jealousy, others are spying on the patient, etc)

Systematized vs nonsystematized	
Systematized	Delusions based on false premises are part of an organized group of delusions. The patient constructs a complex set of delusions to support one or more core delusions
Nonsystematized	Delusions are not related to one another
Delusional themes	
Grandiose	Patient has special significance or powers
Paranoid	Patient is being persecuted, followed, or threatened in some way
Somatic	Patient's body or appearance is viewed as being injured or abnormal in some way
Religious	Patient falsely believes to be in direct or indirect communication with God or a supernatural force, or possessed by a supernatural force; must be atypical of culture, faith or family
Erotomanic/ sexual	Patient falsely believes to have a close, special or sexual relationship with another person
Nihilistic	Bizarre beliefs that one's body is breaking down or that the patient does not really exist
Delusion types	
Of reference	Belief that irrelevant, unrelated or innocuous events in the world have a special personal significance
Of thought	Delusions of thought are referred to as "first-rank" symptoms because their presence is highly suggestive of schizophrenia: • Thought insertion: Thoughts are not one's own but are being inserted from a remote source • Thought withdrawal: Thoughts are being removed by an outside agency • Thought blocking: Long pauses in the middle of expressing a thought, may be blamed on thought withdrawal. Patient usually resumes train of thought on an entirely different topic • Thought broadcasting: Belief that one's thoughts are being passively and continuously broadcast and available to others

2.1.3 Thought Disorganization

These are **impaired, poorly organized and illogical thought processes** that include tangentiality, circumstantiality, derailment, incoherence, thought blocking, clanging, echolalia, and neologisms.

Thought disorganization is a prominent feature of the disorganized type of schizophrenia. Behaviors suggestive of thought disorders are listed in the table below.

Thought Disorders	
Loosening of associations (derailment)	Lack of connection between ideas; jumping from one to another unrelated thought in rapid sequence.
Word salad	Random words arranged into phrases that apparently gives them meaning, but actually carry no significance.
Tangentiality	Excessive digression or deviation from one topic under discussion to other associated but irrelevant topics that arise in the course of a conversation
Circumstantiality	Speech that is highly detailed and very delayed at reaching its goal. Patient may speak about many concepts related to the point of the conversation before eventually returning to the point and concluding the thought.
Flight of ideas	A sequence of loose associations or extreme tangentiality where the speaker goes quickly from one idea to another seemingly unrelated idea. To the listener, the ideas seem unrelated and do not seem to repeat
Perseveration	The repetition of a particular response such as a word, phrase, or gesture despite the absence of the stimulus.
Echolalia	Echoing of one's or other people's speech that may only be committed once, or may be continuous in repetition. This may involve repeating only the last few words or last word of the examiner's sentences.
Neologisms	Words invented by the psychotic person that only have meaning to that person
Clang association	A mode of speech characterized by association of words based upon sound rather than meaning or concepts.
Blocking	Interruption of train of speech before completion, eg, "Am I early?" "No, you're just about on..." (silence)

2.2 Epidemiology of Schizophrenia

- The overall worldwide prevalence of schizophrenia is 1%.
- A higher incidence of schizophrenia is seen among the urban poor, possibly caused by a drift of chronically disabled patients towards poor urban areas

2.2.1 Age of Onset

- Males manifest the illness earlier (ages 18–25) than females (ages 26–45)
- 20% of cases occur after the age of 40 years.

2.2.2 Stress

Stress does not by itself cause schizophrenia, but may affect its onset in predisposed persons, or the recurrence of acute episodes in schizophrenic patients.

2.2.3 Gender Differences

- The lifetime risk of schizophrenia is approximately equal for males and females
- Males experience an earlier age of onset and tend to be more symptomatic

2.2.4 Prenatal Factors

- Obstetric prenatal complications are associated with an increased risk for the child to develop schizophrenia later in life. Fetal stressors that may be involved include hypoxia, fetal malnourishment, or exposure to intrauterine infections
- Winter birth has been associated with an increased risk of developing schizophrenia. The exact cause for this link is unknown, but it may be related to prenatal exposure to viruses such as influenza that are more prevalent during the winter season

2.2.5 Socioeconomic Factors

- Increased prevalence among lower social class, particularly in urban settings
- The two leading theories for this association include the "breeder hypothesis" - higher incidence related to precipitation of onset in susceptible individuals due to urban stressors such as high crime, lack of social cohesion, overstimulation, cramped living spaces, and the "drift hypothesis" - selective migration results in a concentration of schizophrenic people in urban settings
- Studies that studied associations between paternal occupation (as a measure of socioeconomic status at birth) and schizophrenia, have shown an increased risk only for very low socioeconomic births
- Increased prevalence in urban versus rural settings, especially for males

2.2.6 Mortality

- Between 4% and 10% of schizophrenic patients commit suicide
- Mortality due to homicides and violence, as well as medical conditions such as cardiovascular and respiratory disorders, is also higher in this population

2.3   Etiology

- The etiology of schizophrenia is multifactorial and complex, and is thought to include both genetic and environmental factors
- Proposed etiologic factors include dopamine pathway abnormalities (dopamine hypothesis), abnormal reactions to environmental stress (diathesis-stress model), neurodevelopmental abnormalities, and other structural and functional brain changes

2.3.1   Genetics

- Schizophrenia has a strong genetic component, and the degree of risk is proportional to the degree of shared genes. A number of family studies, including twin and adoptive studies, have demonstrated a strong heritable component in schizophrenia
- The concordance rate in monozygotic twins is approx. 50%
- The risk of schizophrenia is increased approx. 10-fold if a parent is affected, and approx. 9-fold if a sibling is affected
- The underlying genetic predisposition is unlikely to be related to abnormalities in a single gene. A number of different chromosomal regions have been consistently implicated by linkage studies
- Candidate genes currently under investigation for involvement in schizophrenia include the neuregulin-1 (NRG1) gene, involved in neurodevelopment and plasticity, and NOS1AP, a gene involved in intracellular nitric oxide regulation
- Some developmental disorders, such as velocardiofacial syndrome, are associated with high rates of schizophrenia

2.3.2   Environmental Factors

As suggested by monozygotic twin studies, genetics are only part of the story, and there is sufficient evidence to suggest that environmental factors play a significant role in the development of schizophrenia.

- Fetal neurodevelopment represents an especially vulnerable period - stressors during this period may predispose the fetus to subsequent development of schizophrenia (see below)
- Exposure to psychoactive drugs in adolescence and young adulthood is associated with increased risk
- Advanced paternal age is more prevalent in schizophrenia than in the general population

2.3.3   Complications of Pregnancy

Several studies have found a higher than average incidence of obstetric and perinatal complications in patients with schizophrenia, suggesting that insults during fetal neurodevelopment play a role in its genesis. These include:
- First or second trimester exposure to viruses or toxins, or fetal starvation
- Perinatal anoxia, birth trauma and exposure to toxins

2.3.4   Neurochemical Factors

Classical Dopamine Hypothesis

The most influential and plausible neurochemical hypothesis is based on the supposed disruption in dopamine neurotransmission in the brain. Evidence for the dopamine hypothesis includes:
- Antipsychotic drugs exercise their effects through the blocking of dopamine action in the brain
- Dopamine-releasing drugs (amphetamine, mescaline, diethyl amide of lysergic acid [LSD]) can induce a state closely resembling paranoid schizophrenia
- Psychotic symptoms are related to dopaminergic hyperactivity in the brain. Hyperactivity of dopaminergic systems during schizophrenia is a result of increased sensitivity and density of dopamine D2 receptors in various parts of the brain

Serotonin Dysfunction

Serotonergic dysfunction is also thought to play a role in schizophrenia. Evidence for this includes:
- The hallucinogen LSD is a 5-HT agonist
- It has been found that in schizophrenia, there are reduced numbers of 5-HT2A receptors and an increase in the number of HT1A receptors in the frontal cortex.
- There are widespread and complex changes in the 5-HT system in schizophrenic patients

Other Neurotransmitters
- **GABA:** Reduced GABA receptors in the hippocampus
- **Glutamate:** Excess glutamate receptors in frontal cortex in postmodern studies. Hypothesis of decreased glutamatergic inhibition of subcortical and mesiotemporal dopamine neurons
- Possible abnormalities of cholecystokinin (CCK)

2.4   The Acute Symptoms of Schizophrenia

The acute symptoms of schizophrenia are divided into two general categories: positive and negative symptoms. These symptoms appear during the acute phase of schizophrenia and are required for a diagnosis of schizophrenia.

- **Positive symptoms (psychosis):** Psychotic symptoms include delusions, hallucinations, and disorganized speech, behavior and thought
- **Negative symptoms (affective and emotional disruption):** Affective symptoms include flattening of affect, avolition, alogia, low energy and motivation, and catatonia

Although not required for diagnosis, other physical manifestations commonly associated with schizophrenia include:

- Mood disorders: Depression and anxiety disorders
- Neurological deficits: Sensory deficits or problems with coordination
- Cognitive impairment: Poor memory, lowered IQ
- Metabolic disorders: Hyperglycemia, hyperlipidemia, hypertension

2.4.1   Positive Symptoms

The term "positive symptoms" in schizophrenia means psychotic symptoms

- These include hallucinations, delusions and disorganized speech, behavior or thought, as described earlier. The most common hallucinations in schizophreniaare auditory hallucinations (40%–80% of patients), usually of an unintelligible or persecutory nature. Hallucinations are a particularly prominent feature of paranoid shizophrenia.
- The delusions of schizophrenia may be quite bizarre, depending on the type, but may not be obvious and require careful questioning to elicit. Delusions of thought (eg, though insertion, withdrawal, broadcasting) are highly suggestive of schizophrenia and are almost pathognomonic.
- Disorganized thinking is also a prominent feature of schizophrenia, particularly of the disorganized (DSM-IV) or hebephrenic (ICD-10) types. Thinking may be so disorganized as to lead to incoherent speech and extremely dysfunctional or bizarre behavior.

2.4.2   Negative Symptoms

- The term "negative symptoms" refers to affective abnormalities and behavioral slowness or rigidity. These are typically prominent features of the disorganized schizophrenia type, and are often present during its residual and prodromal phases.
- Typical negative symptoms include affective flattening (blunted affect, lack of discernible facial emotion, poor eye contact, lack or body movements).

Other negative symptoms include:
– Thought blocking
– Poverty of speech (alogia)
– Poverty of movement (avolition)
– Poverty of joy (anhedonia)

2.4.3   Catatonic Symptoms

- Catatonic symptoms are the prominent feature of the catatonic type of schizophrenia. They can manifest with significant psychomotor disturbances that can either involve excessive excitement or significant immobility
- Catatonic symptoms can also develop as a consequence of a medical illness such as delirium, meningitis, or mood disorders (eg, major depressive disorder or bipolar 1 disorder with catatonic features)

2.5   Phases of Schizophrenia

Although demarcations are not always clear, schizophrenia typically progresses through a series of phases that have been described as follows:

- Premorbid phase
- Prodromal phase
- Acute phase
- Residual phase
- Relapse phase

2.5.1   Premorbid Phase

- Phase is critically important as a potential marker for the future development of schizophrenia
- The Premorbid Assessment Scale (PAS) is a measure of progression of deterioration during the premorbid phase[1]
- Phase is not addressed in the DSM IV

Multiple impairments are evident during the premorbid phase:

- Deficits in cognitive functioning (lower IQ, difficulty in sequencing complex tasks)
- Neurological soft signs (alterations of smooth pursuit eye movements, poor overall motor coordination, impaired sensory integration, decreased ability to recognize objects by touch and feel or to complete finger/thumb position)
- Prominent negative symptomatology is associated with a poorer prognosis
- Odd or unusual personality traits (schizoid), avoidant, and paranoid personality (often termed the premorbid personality)
- Delayed developmental milestones including withdrawal from friends or family or having difficulty showing warmth and developing intimacy
- Certain physical attributes such as a cleft palate, a long face, heart problems, and speech disturbances may be indicative of velocardiofacial syndrome, a complex syndrome significantly associated with schizophrenia

2.5.2   Prodromal Phase

Introduction

- Prodromal phase precedes the onset of acute symptoms, may last from days to years, and may present with attenuated positive and/or negative symptoms.
- A prodromal phase is observed in 75% of schizophrenic patients

Symptoms of Prodromal Phase

Symptoms of prodromal phase include a feeling of tension, poor concentration and difficulty maintaining attention, sleep disorders, depressed mood, poor functioning at work or school or in personal relationships, withdrawal from family and friends, eccentric ideas or erratic behavior. These are further categorized in the table below:

Attenuated Positive Symptoms	Negative Symptoms	Cognitive Symptoms	General Symptoms
• Unusual perception • Odd beliefs/ magical thinking • Vague elaborate speech or circumstantiality • Suspiciousness • Peculiar thought and speech	• Blunted or inappropriate effect • Amotivation, anergia • Social withdrawal • Poor grooming	• Reduced concentration • Poor attention • Poor initiative	• Poor hygiene • Depressed mood • Irritability and anxiety • Poor sleep • Deterioration in functioning
Source: Young and McGorry et al, 1996			

Differential Diagnosis

- Major depression with psychosis
- Schizotypal personality disorder →135
- Borderline personality disorder →137
- Pervasive developmental disorder
- Post Traumatic Stress Disorder (PTSD)
- Obsessive Compulsive Disorder (OCD)
- Attention Deficit Hyperactivity Disorder (ADHD)

Structured Interview For Prodromal Symptoms (SIPS) - A 4 Part Interview

1. Scale Of Prodromal Symptoms (SOPS) (McGlashan et al, 2001)
   - Positive symptoms
   - Negative symptoms
   - Disorganization
   - General symptoms
2. Global Assessment of Functioning (GAF)
3. Schizotypal personality disorder criteria
4. Family history of psychotic illness

The following 5 features are most predictive of progression to schizophrenia based on SIPS (Cannon et al., 2008):
1. Genetic risk with recent deterioration in function
2. Higher levels of unusual thought content
3. Higher levels of suspicion and paranoia
4. Greater social impairment
5. History of substance abuse

Comprehensive Assessment At Risk Mental States (CAARMS)- 3 Part Interview

1. Presence of at least 1 attenuated psychotic symptom
2. Evidence of at least 1 episode of Brief Limited Psychotic Symptoms (BLIPS)
3. Functional decline in past year and genetic risk (one relative with schizotypal personality disorder or psychotic illness)

SIPS and CAARMS scales have high positive predictive value (Young et al., 1996).

Laboratory Diagnosis in the Prodromal Phase

- No specific laboratory or biological markers
- Diagnosis is mostly clinical
- SIPS and CAARMS have high predictive value

Prodromal Treatment[2]

- Use of antipsychotic drugs during the prodromal phase is still under investigation and is NOT at present indicated
- Active follow-up
- Supportive and family therapy
- Education
- Review and monitoring of safety issues
- Treat comorbid conditions if present

2.5.3 Acute Phase

The acute phase is characterized by full-blown symptoms that include hallucinations, delusions, grossly disorganized behavior, disorganized speech or catatonic behavior. These symptoms were described earlier in greater detail. Patient behavior may become so extreme or bizarre that hospitalization is necessary to prevent injury to self or others.

2.5.4 Residual Phase

The residual phase is a period of relative decrease in symptom manifestation between acute phases. Such residual phases are common during the waxing-and-waning course of schizophrenia.

2.5.5 Relapse Phase

The relapse phase describes a return of active phase symptoms following a residual phase and is more common in the paranoid type of schizophrenia. Reasons for relapse are poor medication compliance, substance abuse and stress.

2.6 Diagnostic Classification and Guidelines

This section contains diagnostic classification and criteria information for schizophrenia and other psychotic disorders, or disorders with psychotic features. Both the ICD-10 and DSM-IV-TR classifications and alphanumerical codes are provided, however, the diagnostic information emphasizes the ICD-10 diagnostic guidelines.

The titles of the diagnostic criteria tables contain the ICD-10 numerical codes in parentheses. For reference, whenever a condition subtype has an equivalent DSM-IV-TR classification, the DSM-IV-TR numerical code is also given for that condition (a dash is shown if there is no equivalent classification). However, note that although conditions may have the same name, and include both ICD-10 and DSM-IV-TR codes, the diagnostic criteria used in these two frameworks may be different. Also note that in some cases, the names of mostly equivalent ICD-10 and DSM-IV diagnostic subtypes do not exactly match (eg, the ICD-10 subtype of acute schizophrenia-like psychotic disorder is basically equivalent with the DSM-IV subtype of schizophreniform disorder). For exact DSM-IV criteria, please refer to the latest version of the DSM-IV.

2.6.1 Classification of Schizophrenia

ICD-10 Classification of Schizophrenia (F20)			
Subtype descriptors		**Course descriptors**	
F20.0	Paranoid schizophrenia	F20.x0	Continuous
F20.1	Hebephrenic schizophrenia	F20.x1	Episodic with progressive deficit
F20.2	Catatonic schizophrenia	F20.x2	Episodic with stable deficit
F20.3	Undifferentiated schizophrenia	F20.x3	Episodic remittent
F20.4	Post-schizophrenic depression	F20.x4	Incomplete remission
F20.5	Residual schizophrenia	F20.x5	Complete remission
F20.6	Simple schizophrenia	F20.x6	Other
F20.8	Other schizophrenia	F20.x9	Course uncertain, period of observation too short
F20.9	Schizophrenia, unspecified		

DSM-IV-TR Classification of Schizophrenia (295.xx)	
295.10	Schizophrenia, disorganized type
295.20	Schizophrenia, catatonic type
295.30	Schizophrenia, paranoid type
295.40	Schizophreniform disorder
295.60	Schizophrenia, residual type
295.70	Schizoaffective disorder
295.90	Schizophrenia, undifferentiated type

2.6.2 Classification of Other Psychotic Disorders

ICD-10 Classification of Other Psychotic Disorders	
F21	**Schizotypal disorder**
F22	**Persistent delusional disorder**
F22.0	Delusional disorder
F22.8	Other persistent delusional disorders
F22.9	Persistent delusional disorder, unspecified
F23	**Acute and transient psychotic disorders**
F23.0	Acute polymorphic psychotic disorder without symptoms of schizophrenia
F23.1	Acute polymorphic psychotic disorder with symptoms of schizophrenia
F23.2	Acute schizophrenia-like psychotic disorder
F23.3	Other acute predominantly delusional psychotic disorder

ICD-10 Classification of Other Psychotic Disorders	
F23.8	Other acute and transient psychotic disorders
F23.9	Acute and transient psychotic disorder, unspecified
F23.x0	Without associated acute stress (course descriptor)
F23.x1	With associated acute stress (course descriptor)
F24	**Induced delusional disorder**
F25	**Schizoaffective disorders**
F25.0	Schizoaffective disorder, manic type
F25.1	Schizoaffective disorder, depressive type
F25.2	Schizoaffective disorder, mixed type
F25.8	Other schizoaffective disorders
F25.9	Schizoaffective disorder, unspecified
F28	**Other nonorganic delusional disorders**
F29	**Unspecified nonorganic psychosis**

DSM-IV-TR Classification of Other Psychotic Disorders or Features	
290.42	Vascular dementia, with delusions
291.3	Alcohol-induced psychotic disorder, with hallucinations
291.5	Alcohol-induced psychotic disorder, with delusions
292.11	Substance-induced psychotic disorder, with delusions*
292.12	Substance-induced psychotic disorder, with hallucinations*
293.81	Psychotic disorder due to general medical condition, with delusions*
293.82	Psychotic disorder due to general medical condition, with hallucinations*
296.24	Major depressive disorder, single episode, severe with psychotic features
296.34	Major depressive disorder, recurrent, severe with psychotic features
296.04	Bipolar I disorder, single manic episode, severe with psychotic features
296.44	Bipolar I disorder, most recent episode manic, severe with psychotic features
296.54	Bipolar I disorder, most recent episode depressed, severe with psychotic features
296.64	Bipolar I disorder, most recent episode mixed, severe with psychotic features
297.1	Delusional disorder
297.3	Shared psychotic disorder
298.8	Brief psychotic disorder
298.9	Psychotic disorder NOS
*Specify the medical condition or substance associated with the psychotic condition.	

2.6.3 Schizophrenia, General

Schizophrenia (F20, 295.x)	
Prototypical Symptoms per ICD-10	
a.	Thought echo, thought insertion or withdrawal, and thought broadcasting
b.	Delusions of control, influence, or passivity, clearly referred to body or limb movements or specific thoughts, actions, or sensations; delusional perception
c.	Hallucinatory voices giving a running commentary on the patient's behavior, or discussing the patient among themselves, or other types of hallucinatory voices coming from some part of the body
d.	Persistent delusions of other kinds that are culturally inappropriate and completely impossible, such as religious or political identity, or superhuman powers and abilities (eg, being able to control the weather, or being in communication with aliens from another world)
e.	Persistent hallucinations in any modality, when accompanied either by fleeting or half-formed delusions without clear affective content, or by persistent over-valued ideas, or when occurring every day for weeks or months on end
f.	Breaks or interpolations in the train of thought, resulting in incoherence or irrelevant speech, or neologisms
g.	Catatonic behavior, such as excitement, posturing, or waxy flexibility, negativism, mutism, and stupor
h.	Negative symptoms such as marked apathy, paucity of speech, and blunting or incongruity of emotional responses, usually resulting in social withdrawal and lowering of social performance; it must be clear that these are not due to depression or to neuroleptic medication
i.	A significant and consistent change in the overall quality of some aspects of personal behavior, manifest as loss of interest, aimlessness, idleness, a self-absorbed attitude, and social withdrawal
ICD-10 Diagnostic Guidelines	
• A minimum of **1 very clear symptom** (or 2 or more if less clear-cut) from symptom **groups a–d** OR **symptoms from at least 2 of the symptom groups e–h** clearly present for most of the time during **a period of 1 month or more.** • If duration < 1 month, diagnose as acute schizophrenia-like psychotic disorder; reclassify as schizophrenia if duration longer than 1 month • Symptom group(i) in the above list applies only to the diagnosis of Simple Schizophrenia (F20.6), and a duration of at least one year is required.	
Diagnostic Exclusions	

Schizophrenia (F20, 295.x)

- The diagnosis should not be made in the presence of extensive depressive or manic symptoms unless it is clear that schizophrenic symptoms antedated the affective disturbance.
- If both schizophrenic and affective symptoms develop together and are evenly balanced, the diagnosis of schizoaffective disorder (F25.-) should be made, even if the schizophrenic symptoms by themselves would have justified the diagnosis of schizophrenia.
- Schizophrenia should not be diagnosed in the presence of overt brain disease or during states of drug intoxication or withdrawal.
- Similar disorders developing in the presence of epilepsy or other brain disease should be coded under F06.2 and those induced by drugs under F1x.5.

DSM-IV Diagnosis of Schizophrenia (295.xx)

According to the DSM-IV, the diagnosis of schizophrenia requires at least 2 characteristic positive or negative symptoms, as follows:

- Significant symptom duration in any 1 month period (less if effectively treated)
- Symptoms persist for at least 6 months that may contain relatively asymptomatic or mildly symptomatic periods, but at least 1 month of continuous symptoms
- Significant social or occupational impairment
- Other causes of psychosis have been ruled out (eg, severe mood disorder, substance abuse, medical conditions, etc)

For exact diagnostic criteria please refer to the DSM IV-TR.

2.6.4 Paranoid Schizophrenia

Paranoid Schizophrenia (F20.0, 295.30)

Prototypical Symptoms per ICD-10

- Delusions of persecution, reference, exalted birth, special mission, bodily change, or jealousy
- Hallucinatory voices that threaten the patient or give commands, or auditory hallucinations without verbal form, such as whistling, humming, or laughing
- Hallucinations of smell or taste, or of sexual or other bodily sensations; visual hallucinations may occur but are rarely predominant

ICD-10 Diagnostic Guidelines

- The general criteria for a diagnosis of schizophrenia must be satisfied
- **Hallucinations and/or delusions must be prominent**. Delusions can be of almost any kind, but delusions of control, influence, or passivity, and persecutory beliefs of various kinds are the most characteristic
- Negative symptoms, disturbances of affect, volition and speech, and catatonic symptoms must be relatively inconspicuous

Paranoid Schizophrenia (F20.0, 295.30)
Diagnostic Exclusions

- Exclude epileptic and drug-induced psychoses
- Persecutory delusions might carry little diagnostic weight in people from certain countries or cultures

2.6.5   Hebephrenic Schizophrenia

Hebephrenic Schizophrenia (F20.1, -)
Prototypical Symptoms per ICD-10

- Prominent negative symptoms and affective changes, fleeting and fragmentary delusions and hallucinations, irresponsible and unpredictable behavior and mannerisms; hallucinations and delusions may be present but are not prominent
- Shallow and inappropriate mood often accompanied by giggling or self-satisfied, self-absorbed smiling, or by a lofty manner, grimaces, mannerisms, pranks, hypochondriacal complaints, and reiterated phrases
- Disorganized thought, rambling and incoherent speech
- Tendency to remain solitary, behavior seems empty of purpose and feeling
- Loss of drive and determination, goal abandonment
- A superficial and manneristic preoccupation with religion, philosophy, and other abstract themes

ICD-10 Diagnostic Guidelines

- The general criteria for a diagnosis of schizophrenia must be satisfied
- Should normally be diagnosed for the first time only in adolescents or young adults (15-20 years)
- **A period of 2 or 3 months** of continuous observation is usually necessary

2.6.6   Catatonic Schizophrenia

Catatonic Schizophrenia (F20.2, 295.20)
Prototypical Symptoms per ICD-10

a.	Stupor (marked decrease in reactivity to the environment and in spontaneous movements and activity) or mutism
b.	Excitement (apparently purposeless motor activity, not influenced by external stimuli)
c.	Posturing (voluntary assumption and maintenance of inappropriate or bizarre postures)
d.	Negativism (an apparently motiveless resistance to all instructions or attempts to be moved, or movement in the opposite direction)
e.	Rigidity (maintenance of a rigid posture against efforts to be moved)

Catatonic Schizophrenia (F20.2, 295.20)	
Prototypical Symptoms per ICD-10 (cont.)	
f.	Waxy flexibility (maintenance of limbs and body in externally imposed positions)
g.	Other symptoms such as command automatism (automatic compliance with instructions), and perseveration of words and phrases
ICD-10 Diagnostic Guidelines	
• The general criteria for a diagnosis of schizophrenia must be satisfied	
• Requires that **1 or more of the prototypical catatonic symptoms in a–g** dominate the clinical picture	
Diagnostic Exclusions	
• Rule out brain diseases, metabolic disturbances, alcohol or drugs, and mood disorders	

2.6.7 Undifferentiated Schizophrenia

Undifferentiated Schizophrenia (F20.3, 295.90)
ICD-10 Diagnostic Guidelines
• Disoder meets the general criteria for schizophrenia
• Disorder is either without sufficient symptoms to meet the criteria for only one of the subtypes F20.0, F20.1, F20.2, F20.4, or F20.5, or with so many symptoms that the criteria for more than one of the paranoid (F20.0), hebephrenic (F20.1), or catatonic (F20.2) subtypes are met

2.6.8 Post-Schizophrenic Depression

Post-Schizophrenic Depression (F20.4, –)
ICD-10 Diagnostic Guidelines
• The patient has had a schizophrenic illness meeting the general criteria for **schizophrenia within the past 12 months**
• Some schizophrenic symptoms (positive or negative) are still present; and
• Depressive symptoms are prominent and distressing, fulfilling at least the criteria for a depressive episode (F32.-), and have been present for **at least 2 weeks.**

2.6.9   Residual Schizophrenia

Residual Schizophrenia (F20.5, 295.60)

ICD-10 Diagnostic Guidelines

- **Prominent negative schizophrenic symptoms,** ie, psychomotor slowing, underactivity, blunting of affect, passivity and lack of initiative, poverty of quantity or content of speech, poor nonverbal communication by facial expression, eye contact, voice modulation, and posture, poor self-care and social performance
- Evidence in the past of **at least 1 clear-cut psychotic episode** meeting the diagnostic criteria for schizophrenia
- A **period of at least 1 year** during which the intensity and frequency of florid symptoms such as delusions and hallucinations have been minimal or substantially reduced and the negative schizophrenic syndrome has been present
- Absence of dementia or other organic brain disease or disorder, and of chronic depression or institutionalism sufficient to explain the negative impairments

2.6.10   Simple Schizophrenia

Simple Schizophrenia (F20.6, -)

Prototypical Symptoms per ICD-10

- Insidious but progressive development of oddities of conduct, inability to meet the demands of society, and decline in total performance
- Delusions and hallucinations are not evident, and the disorder is less obviously psychotic than the hebephrenic, paranoid, and catatonic subtypes of schizophrenia
- The characteristic negative features of residual schizophrenia (eg, blunting of affect, loss of volition) develop without being preceded by any overt psychotic symptoms
- With increasing social impoverishment, vagrancy may ensue and the individual may then become self-absorbed, idle, and aimless

ICD-10 Diagnostic Guidelines

- Significant changes in personal behavior, manifest as a marked loss of interest, idleness, and social withdrawal over a period of **at least 1 year**
- Slowly progressive development of the characteristic negative symptoms of residual schizophrenia (see F20.5) without any history of hallucinations, delusions, or other manifestations of an earlier psychotic episode

2.6.11 Schizotypal Disorder

Schizotypal Disorder (F21, –)

Prototypical Symptoms per ICD-10

- Inappropriate or constricted affect (the individual appears cold and aloof)
- Behaviour or appearance that is odd, eccentric, or peculiar
- Poor rapport with others and a tendency to social withdrawal
- Odd beliefs or magical thinking, influencing behavior and inconsistent with subcultural norms
- Suspiciousness or paranoid ideas
- Obsessive ruminations without inner resistance, often with dysmorphophobic, sexual or aggressive contents
- Unusual perceptual experiences including somatosensory (bodily) or other illusions, depersonalization or derealization
- Vague, circumstantial, metaphorical, overelaborate, or stereotyped thinking, manifested by odd speech or in other ways, without gross incoherence
- Occasional transient quasipsychotic episodes with intense illusions, auditory or other hallucinations, and delusion-like ideas, usually occurring without external provocation

ICD-10 Diagnostic Guidelines

- **3-4 of the typical features** listed above should have been present, continuously or episodically, for **at least 2 years**
- The individual must never have met criteria for schizophrenia itself
- A history of schizophrenia in a first-degree relative gives additional weight to the diagnosis but is not a prerequisite

2.6.12 Persistent Delusional Disorders

Delusional Disorder (F22.0, 297.1)

Prototypical Symptoms per ICD-10

- Characterized by the development either of a single delusion or of a set of related delusions which are usually persistent and sometimes lifelong
- Delusions are typically persecutory, hypochondriacal, or grandiose, but they may be concerned with litigation or jealousy, or express a conviction that the individual's body is misshapen, or that others think that he or she smells or is homosexual
- Depressive symptoms may be present intermittently, and olfactory and tactile hallucinations may develop in some cases; occasional or transitory auditory hallucinations, particularly in elderly patients, do not rule out this diagnosis, provided that they are not typically schizophrenic and form only a small part of the overall clinical picture
- Onset is commonly in middle age but sometimes, particularly in the case of beliefs about having a misshapen body, in early adult life

Delusional Disorder (F22.0, 297.1)

ICD-10 Diagnostic Guidelines

- Delusions **must be present for at least 3 months**
- Delusions must be clearly personal rather than subcultural
- Delusions must constitute the most conspicuous or the only clinical characteristic

Diagnostic Exclusions

- Clear and persistent auditory hallucinations (voices), schizophrenic symptoms such as delusions of control and marked blunting of affect, and definite evidence of brain disease are all incompatible with this diagnosis

Other Persistent Delusional Disorders (F22.8, –)

ICD-10 Diagnostic Guidelines

- Persistent delusional disorders **lasting longer than 3 months** that do not meet the criteria for delusional disorder (F22.0)
- Disorders in which delusions are accompanied by persistent hallucinatory voices or by schizophrenic symptoms that are insufficient to meet criteria for schizophrenia (F20.–)

2.6.13 Acute and Transient Psychotic Disorders

Acute and Transient Psychotic Disorders (F23, 298.8)*

ICD-10 Diagnostic Guidelines

- Psychotic symptoms develop **within 2 weeks** or less; if developing within 48 hours or less, abrupt onset should be specified
- The presence of typical syndromes such as typical schizophrenic symptoms or polymorphic psychotic symptoms

ICD-10 Subtypes

With Associated Acute Stress (F23.x0)

- Associated with the presence of culturally appropriate acute stress such as bereavement, unexpected loss of partner or job, marriage, or the psychological trauma of combat, terrorism, and torture; long-standing difficulties or problems should not be included as a source of stress in this context

Without associated acute stress (F23.x1)

- Not associated with identifiable acute stress factors

Diagnostic Exclusions

- Does not satisfy the criteria for manic or depressive episodes
- Organic causes such as concussion, dementia or delirium
- Drug or alcohol intoxication

*The DSM-IV classifies this as Brief Psychotic Disorder (298.8).

2.6.14 Acute Polymorphic Psychotic Disorder

Acute Polymorphic Psychotic Disorder (F23.x, -)

Prototypical Symptoms per ICD-10

- Acute psychotic disorder in which hallucinations, delusions, and perceptual disturbances are obvious but markedly variable, changing from day to day or even from hour to hour
- Emotional turmoil, with intense transient feelings of happiness and ecstasy or anxieties and irritability, is frequently present
- Particularly likely to have an abrupt onset (within 48 hours) and a rapid resolution of symptoms
- In a large proportion of cases there is no obvious precipitating stress

ICD-10 Diagnostic Guidelines

- **Acute onset (within less than 2 weeks)** and **duration less than 3 months**
- There must be several types of hallucination or delusion, changing in both type and intensity from day to day or within the same day
- There should be a similarly varying emotional state

ICD-10 Subtypes

Without symptoms of schizophrenia (F23.0)

- None of the symptoms are present with sufficient consistency to fulfill the criteria for schizophrenia (F20.-) or for manic or depressive episode (F30.- or F32.-)
- Persistent delusional disorder (F22.-) or other nonorganic psychotic disorder (F28) is likely to be the most appropriate if duration is longer than 3 months

With symptoms of schizophrenia (F23.1)

- Typically schizophrenic symptoms are also consistently present, but for **less than 1 month**
- If the schizophrenia symptoms persist for longer than 1 month, the diagnosis should be changed to schizophrenia

2.6.15 Acute Schizophrenia-like Psychotic Disorder

Acute Schizophrenia-like Psychotic Disorder (F23.2, 295.40)*

ICD-10 Diagnostic Guidelines

- The onset of psychotic symptoms must be acute (**2 weeks or less** from a nonpsychotic to a clearly psychotic state), but the **duration is less than 1 month**
- Symptoms that fulfill the criteria for schizophrenia (F20.-) must have been present for the majority of the time since the establishment of an obviously psychotic clinical picture
- The criteria for acute polymorphic psychotic disorder (F23) are not fulfilled

Diagnostic Exclusions

- If the schizophrenic symptoms last for more than 1 month, the diagnosis should be changed to schizophrenia (F20.-)

*The DSM-IV classifies this as Schizophreniform Disorder (295.40).

2.6.16 Other Psychotic Disorders

Other Acute Predominantly Delusional Psychotic Disorders (F23,3, -)

Prototypical Symptoms per ICD-10

- Acute psychotic disorders in which comparatively stable delusions or hallucinations are the main clinical features, but do not fulfill the criteria for schizophrenia (F20.-).
- Delusions of persecution or reference are common, and hallucinations are usually auditory (voices talking directly to the patient)

ICD-10 Diagnostic Guidelines

- The onset of psychotic symptoms must be acute (**2 weeks or less** from a nonpsychotic to a clearly psychotic state), and **duration is less than 3 months**
- Delusions or hallucinations must have been present for the majority of the time since the establishment of an obviously psychotic state; and
- The criteria for neither schizophrenia (F20.-) nor acute polymorphic psychotic disorder (F23.0) are fulfilled

Other Acute and Transient Psychotic Disorders (F23.8, -)

ICD-10 Diagnostic Guidelines

- Any other acute psychotic disorders that are unclassifiable under any other category in F23 (such as acute psychotic states in which definite delusions or hallucinations occur but persist for only small proportions of the time)
- States of undifferentiated excitement if more detailed information about the patient's mental state is not available

Diagnostic Exclusions

- Organic causes

2.6.17 Induced Delusional Disorder

Induced Delusional Disorder (F24, 297.3)*

ICD-10 Diagnostic Guidelines
- A delusional disorder shared by two or more people with close emotional links
- Only one of the people suffers from a genuine psychotic disorder; the delusions are induced in the other(s) and usually disappear when the people are separated

*The DSM-IV classifies this as Shared Psychotic Disorder (297.3).

2.6.18 Schizoaffective Disorders, General

Schizoaffective Disorders (F25, 295.70)*

ICD-10 Diagnostic Guidelines
- Both definite schizophrenic and definite affective symptoms are prominent simultaneously, or within a few days of each other, within the same episode of illness, and, as a consequence of this, the episode of illness does not meet criteria for either schizophrenia or a depressive or manic episode

Diagnostic Exclusions
- The term should not be applied to patients who exhibit schizophrenic symptoms and affective symptoms only in different episodes of illness

*The DSM-IV does not differentiate between Manic, Depressive or Mixed types of Shizoaffective disorders. All Schizoaffective Disorders are classified as (295.70).

2.6.19 Schizoaffective Disorder, Manic Type

Schizoaffective Disorder, Manic Type (F25.0, 295.70)*

Prototypical Symptoms per ICD-10

a.	The abnormality of mood usually takes the form of elation, accompanied by increased self-esteem and grandiose ideas, but sometimes excitement or irritability are more obvious and accompanied by aggressive behavior and persecutory ideas
b.	Increased energy, overactivity, impaired concentration, and a loss of normal social inhibition
c.	Delusions of reference, grandeur, or persecution may be present, but other more typically schizophrenic symptoms are required to establish the diagnosis (eg, thought broadcasting or interference)

ICD-10 Diagnostic Guidelines
- Must exhibit **prominent elevation of mood,** or a less obvious elevation of mood combined with increased irritability or excitement
- Within the same episode, **at least 1 and preferably 2 typically schizophrenic symptoms** (as specified for schizophrenia (F20.-), diagnostic guidelines (a)-(d)) should be clearly present

*The DSM-IV does not differentiate between Manic, Depressive or Mixed types of Shizoaffective disorders. All Schizoaffective Disorders are classified as (295.70).

2.6.20 Schizoaffective Disorder, Depressive Type

Schizoaffective Disorder, Depressive Type (F25.1, 295.70)*
Prototypical Symptoms per ICD-10
a.	Depression of mood is usually accompanied by several characteristic depressive symptoms or behavioral abnormalities such as retardation, insomnia, loss of energy, appetite or weight, reduction of normal interests, impairment of concentration, guilt, feelings of hopelessness, and suicidal thoughts
b.	At the same time, or within the same episode, other more typically schizophrenic symptoms are present
c.	Schizoaffective episodes of the depressive type are usually less florid and alarming than schizoaffective episodes of the manic type, but they tend to last longer and the prognosis is less favorable
ICD-10 Diagnostic Guidelines
• Prominent depression, accompanied by **at least 2 characteristic depressive symptoms** or associated behavioral abnormalities as listed for depressive episode (F32.-)
• Within the same episode, **at least 1 and preferably 2 typically schizophrenic symptoms** (as specified for schizophrenia (F20.-), diagnostic guidelines (a)-(d)) should be clearly present

*The DSM-IV does not differentiate between Manic, Depressive or Mixed types of Shizoaffective disorders. All Schizoaffective Disorders are classified as (295.70).

2.6.21 Schizoaffective Disorder, Mixed Type

Schizoaffective Disorder, Mixed Type (F25.2, 295.70)*
ICD-10 Diagnostic Guidelines
• Disorders in which symptoms of schizophrenia (F20.-) coexist with those of a mixed bipolar affective disorder (F31.6)

*The DSM-IV does not differentiate between Manic, Depressive or Mixed types of Shizoaffective disorders. All Schizoaffective Disorders are classified as (295.70).

2.6.22 Nonorganic Psychotic Disorders

Other Nonorganic Psychotic Disorders (F28, -)
ICD-10 Diagnostic Guidelines
• Psychotic disorders that do not meet the criteria for schizophrenia (F20.-) or for psychotic types of mood [affective] disorders (F30-F39), and psychotic disorders that do not meet the symptomatic criteria for persistent delusional disorder (F22.-)

Unspecified Nonorganic Psychosis (F29, 298.9)
ICD-10 Diagnostic Guidelines
• This category should be used for psychosis of unknown etiology

*The DSM-IV classifies this as Psychotic Disorder NOS (298.9).

2.7   Differential Diagnosis of Psychotic Symptoms

2.7.1   Axis I Disorders

- Mood disorders
- Acute schizophrenia-like psychotic disorder (schizophreniform disorder)
- Brief reactive psychosis
- Schizotypal personality disorder
- Delusional disorder
- Drug induced psychosis
- Organic etiologies

2.7.2   Axis II Disorders

- Cluster A personality disorders (schizotypal, paranoid, schizoid personality disorder)
- Cluster B disorders
- Borderline Personality Disorder

2.7.3   Axis III Disorders

- Acute confusional stage
- Iatrogenic disorders

2.8   Neuroimaging Findings in Schizophrenia

- Early CT studies have shown nonspecific ventricular enlargement of the cortical sulcal prominence
- PET and MRI studies have shown that frontal and temporal lobes are major sites of abnormalities
- Current evidence favors generalized cortical tissue loss and functional disconnectivity in schizophrenia
- Structural brain abnormalities are subtle but reproducible [3]
- Family members at risk also show similar but more subtle brain changes [4]

2.9 Treatment For Schizophrenia

2.9.1 Overview

Although there are a range of treatments that can control the symptoms of schizophreniaand slow its course, there is presently no cure for this disease and its course is progressive. Treatments are most effective when they involve a combination of pharmacotherapy and psychotherapy in the context of an well-developed social and family support structure.

2.9.2 Treatment Stages

- Treatment of the first psychotic episode and recurrent acute psychosis
- Maintenance treatment
- Treatment of refractory conditions
- Other adjunctive treatments for schizophrenia
- Psychosocial treatments

2.9.3 Treatment Principles

- Pharmacologic treatment
- Individual supportive therapy
- Cognitive and psychosocial therapies
- Family psychoeducation and support
- Social support
- Case management
- Housing
- Financial support
- Vocational support

2.10   Pharmacological Treatment Guidelines

Any stage(s) can be skipped depending on the clinical picture or history of antipsychotic failures.

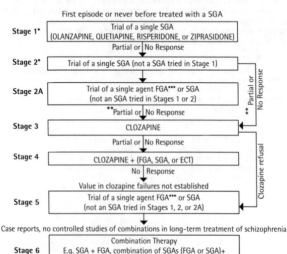

First episode or never before treated with a SGA

Stage 1*
Trial of a single SGA
(OLANZAPINE, QUETIAPINE, RISPERIDONE, or ZIPRASIDONE)

Partial or No Response

Stage 2*
Trial of a single SGA (not a SGA tried in Stage 1)

Stage 2A
Trial of a single agent FGA*** or SGA
(not an SGA tried in Stages 1 or 2)

**Partial or No Response

Stage 3
CLOZAPINE

Partial or No Response

Stage 4
CLOZAPINE + (FGA, SGA, or ECT)

No Response

Value in clozapine failures not established

Stage 5
Trial of a single agent FGA*** or SGA
(not an SGA tried in Stages 1, 2, or 2A)

Partial or No Response

**

Clozapine refusal

Case reports, no controlled studies of combinations in long-term treatment of schizophrenia

Stage 6
Combination Therapy
E.g. SGA + FGA, combination of SGAs (FGA or SGA)+
ECT, (FGA or SGA) + other agent(e.g. mood stabilizer)****

*If patient is nonadherent to medication, the clinician may use haloperidol decanoate or fluphenazine decanoate at any stage, but should carefully assess for unrecognized side effects and consider a different oral AP if side effects could be contributing to nonadherence.
** See original text for discussion. Current expert opinion favors choice of clozapine.
***Assuming no history of failure on FGA.
****Whenever a second medication is added to an antipsychotic (other than clozapine) for the purpose of improving psychotic symptoms, the patient is considered to be in Stage 6.
See Description of Tactics and Critical Decision Points section for more explanation.
AP = Antipsychotic, FGA = First generation AP, SGA = Second generation AP

2.11 Side Effect Management

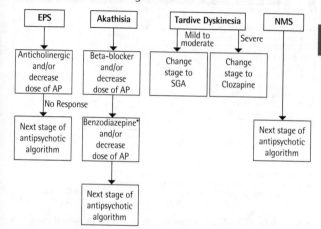

2.12 Characteristics of Antipsychotics

Characteristics of Typical Antipsychotics	Characteristics of Ideal Atypical Antipsychotics
• D2 receptor blockade • High EPS/TD potential • Efficacy limited to positive symptoms • Prolactin elevation • Affect all the dopamine pathways	• Effective for positive and negative symptoms • 5HT2/D2 Blockade • Efficacy across multiple domains • No to low EPS/TD potential • Avoid sustained hyperprolactinemia

Conventional Antipsychotics	Atypical Antipsychotics
• Aliphatic phenothiazine: Chlorpromazine • Piperazine phenothiazines: Perphenazine, trifluoperazine, fluphenazine • Piperidine phenothiazines: Thioridazine, mesoridazine • Thioxanthene: Thiothixene • Dibenzodiazepine: Loxapine • Indolone: Molindone • Butyrophenone: Haloperidol • Diphenylbutylpiperidine: Pimozide	• Aripiprazole • Clozapine • Olanzapine • Paliperidone • Quetiapine • Risperidone • Ziprasidone
EPS = extrapyramidal symptoms, TD = tardive dyskinesia	

2.13 Atypical Antipsychotics

2.13.1 Clozapine

Mechanism of Action

- Clozapine has a wide range of physiological actions
- Clozapine shows high in vitro receptor affinities for the D4, 5HT2 , alpha 1, adrenergic, and muscarinic H1 receptors, and relatively weak affinity for D1, D2 and D3 receptors
- The high 5HT2/D2 ratio is hypothesized to be responsible for many of clozapine's advantages over typical antipsychotic drugs

Side Effects

- Agranulocytosis
- Extrapyramidal side effects
- Sedation
- Cardiovascular effects
- Weight gain
- Endocrine effects
- Hypersalivation
- Fever
- Seizures
- Anticholinergic side effects
- Obsessive compulsive symptoms

2.13.2 Olanzapine

- Olanzapine is based on a modification of the clozapine molecule
- Olanzapine is a monoaminergic antagonist with high affinity for the 5HT2 and D1, D2, D3 and D4 receptors
- Compared with clozapine, olanzapine has greater D2 and weaker D4 and alpha adrenergic affinity
- Despite its structural similarity to clozapine, olanzapine is not associated with a high incidence of agranulocytosis

Clinical Use

- Recommended starting dose of olanzapine is 10 mg at bedtime for schizophrenia and 10-15 mg at bedtime for acutely manic patients

Side Effects

- Somnolence is a common side effect; patients often become tolerant of this side effect over time
- Anticholinergic side effects
- Seizures
- Hepatic effects
- Weight gain

2.13.3 Risperidone

- Risperidone is an atypical antipsychotic medication that combines D2 receptor antagonism with potent 5HT2 receptor antagonism
- Risperidone has higher affinity for D2 receptors than does clozapine
- Risperidone also antagonizes D1 and D4 receptors, alpha 1, and alpha 2 adrenergic receptors and H1 receptors
- Risperidone is most effective at total daily doses of 4-6 mg

Side Effects

- Insomnia, hypotension, agitation, headache and rhinitis are the most common side effects of risperidone. These tend to lessen with time
- Overall, the drug tends to be well tolerated. Risperidone does not have significant anticholinergic side effects
- Hyperprolactinemia is common
- Extrapyramidal side effects
- Cardiovascular effects
- Tardive disorders
- Weight gain

2.13.4 Quetiapine

- Quetiapine has weak affinity for 5HT1A, 5HT2, D1, D2, H1, alpha 1, and alpha 2 receptors
- Quetiapine exhibits very week affinity for D2 receptors
- Quetiapine's selectively high 5HT2/D2 ratio is consistent with its atypical anti psychotic properties
- Antagonism of H1 receptors is associated with sedative side effects and alpha 1 antagonism is associated with orthostatic hypertension

Side Effects

- Somnolence is one of the most common side effects of quetiapine. Somnolence and psychomotor slowing are dose dependant and patients often become tolerant to these side effects over time

Quetiapine Side Effects (cont.)
- Ocular changes
- Cardiovascular effect
- Hepatic effect
- Weight gain

2.13.5 Ziprasidone

Ziprasidone is the only atypical antipsychotic available in capsule form. This medication combines high affinity for 5HT2 receptors with an intermediate affinity for D2 resulting in very high 5HT2/D2 affinity ratio

Side Effects
- Cardiovascular effects
- Weight gain

2.13.6 Aripiprazole

Aripiprazole has higher affinity for D2 and D3 receptors as well as 5HT1A and 5HT2A receptors. Aripiprazole has partial antagonist activity at the D2 and 5HT21A receptors and antagonist activity at the 5HT2A receptor

Side Effects
- Headache, nausea, dyspepsia, agitation, anxiety, insomnia, somnolence and akathisia
- Aripiprazole is not associated with significant sedation, anticholinergic side effects, weight gain or cardiovascular side effects
- As with all other antipsychotic medication, aripiprazole is associated with risk for neuroleptic malignant syndrome and dyskinesias

2.13.7 Paliperidone

- This medication functions as an antagonist at the D2 5HT2A, alpha 1, alpha 2 and H1 receptors
- The risks associated with paliperidone are similar to those for the atypical antipsychotics
- The most common side effects include tachycardia, headache, somnolence, anxiety, extrapyramidal symptoms including Parkinsonism, akathisia, dyskinesia and tremor

2.14 Side Effects of Antipsychotic Medications

Side Effects	Descriptions
Extrapyramidal Symptoms (EPS)	• The pyramidal system is responsible for voluntary movement and the extrapyramidal system is responsible for involuntary muscle action • Drug effects on these systems therefore produce various movement disorders including dystonias, rigidity, Parkinsonism, akathisia & tardive dyskinesia
Acute Dystonia	• Sustained muscular contraction of neck, eyes, throat • Generally occurs soon after starting medication
Akathisia	• Uncomfortable continuous motor restlessness • Can occur at any time during treatment, but generally occur the first few week(s) • Easily misdiagnosed as an underlying psychiatric disorder
Neuroleptic Malignant Syndrome (NMS)	• Pipe-like rigidity, fever, tremor, altered level of consciousness • Hypotension, tachycardia • Laboratory abnormalities- elevated WBC & CK • Mortality 10-20% • Can occur at any time in the course of treatment
Tardive Dyskinesia (TD)	• Spastic facial distortions and tongue movements • May extend to neck, trunk, and extremities • Delayed effect, usually beyond 6 months from starting medication • Increases with duration of exposure to antipsychotic • Known to occur without antipsychotic therapy • May be permanent, occur on discontinuation or resolve on its own • Is worsened by medications used to treat other EPS symptoms
Anticholinergic Symptoms	• Dry mouth, blurred vision, constipation, urinary retention, mydriasis (dilated pupils)

Side Effects (cont.)	Descriptions

Endocrine Effects	• Hyperprolactinemia occurs with drugs that exhibit strong D2 affinity and has the following symptoms:
	  – Women: Amenorrhea/galactorrhea, false-positive pregnancy test results, decreased libido
	  – Men: Decreased libido, erectile dysfunction, gynecomastia
	• Possible association with pancreatitis with some atypicals (especially clozapine and olanzapine)

Sexual Effects	Impotence, infertility, diminished libido
Ocular Effects	Cornea and lens deposits, retinal deposits
Dermatological Effects	Skin eruptions
Cardiac effects	Ventricular arrhythmias, abnormal cardiac conduction, orthostatic (postural) hypotension, tachycardia
Hepatic Effects	Cholestatic jaundice
Hematological Effects	Agranulocytosis (especially with clozapine)
Metabolic Effects	Primarily in 2nd generation atypical antipsychotics • Weight gain • Hyperglycemia • Hyperlipidemia

2.15 Prognosis of Schizophrenia

The rule of thirds: 1/3 - Good prognosis; 1/3 - Intermediate prognosis; 1/3 - Poor prognosis

Predictors of Good Prognosis	Predictors of Poor Prognosis
• Female sex • Good premorbid functioning • Acute onset of symptoms • Presence of precipitating stressors • Predominantly positive symptoms • Predominant mood symptoms • Family history of mood disorders • Insight into having an illness • Good support system • Good response to antipsychotic medication	• Male sex • History of obstetric complications • Abnormal premorbid personality • Low IQ • Single status • Early age at onset • Insidious onset • Substance abuse • Family history of schizophrenia • Predominantly negative symptoms • Disorganized type of schizophrenia • Poor insight into having an illness • Poor support system

List of references

[1] Cannon-Spoor, H. Eleanor, Potkin Steven G, Wyatt; Richard J. Schizophrenia Bulletin
[2] Reference McGorry et al 2005
[3] Shenton et al 2001
[4] Lawrie et al 2002 & Seidman et al 2002

3   Anxiety Disorders

3.1   General Information

Anxiety disorders are characterized by excessive and unwarranted fear, worry, panic and anxiety that is either general and nonspecific in nature, or is triggered by specific situations, environments, or animate or inanimate objects. These feelings are difficult to control and cause significant distress and impairment.

3.1.1   Mental and Physical Manifestations of Anxiety

Physical Symptoms	Affective Symptoms	Behavioral Component	Cognitive Symptoms
Autonomic arousal: • Tachycardia • Palpitations • Tachypnea • Diaphoresis • Diarrhea • Light headedness • Chest pain	• Edginess • Experience of terror • Feelings that one is "going to die" • Feelings that one is "going to lose control" • Subjective apprehension • Feelings of impending death	• Avoidance behavior	• Worry • Apprehension • Obsessions • Thoughts about emotional or bodily damage • Fear

3.1.2   Epidemiology

- An anxiety disorder often begins in early life, but may occur for the first time in middle age
- Anxiety disorders are among the most prevalent and disabling psychiatric condition in the general population
- Women are affected more than men
- 4%-7% prevalence in the normal population
- Anxiety disorders account for 27% of psychiatric consultations in general practice, and 8% of psychiatric outpatient consultations

Prevalence of Anxiety Disorders[5]		
Disorder	**12 Month Prevalence**	**Lifetime Prevalence**
Generalized Anxiety Disorder	3.1	5.7
Panic Disorder	2.7	4.7
Obsessive Compulsive Disorder	1.0	1.6
Posttraumatic Stress Disorder	3.5	6.8
Social Phobia	6.8	12.1

From: Kessler et al. Archives of General Psychiatry 2005.

3.2 Classification

ICD-10 Classification of Anxiety and Stress-Related Disorders	
F40	**Phobic anxiety disorders**
F40.0	Agoraphobia
F40.00	Agoraphobia without panic disorder
F40.01	Agoraphobia with panic disorder
F40.1	Social phobias
F40.2	Specific (isolated) phobias
F40.8	Other phobic anxiety disorders
F40.9	Phobic anxiety disorder, unspecified
F41	**Other anxiety disorders**
F41.0	Panic disorder (episodic paroxysmal anxiety)
F41.1	Generalized anxiety disorder (GAD)
F41.2	Mixed anxiety and depressive disorder
F41.3	Other mixed anxiety disorders
F41.8	Other specified anxiety disorders
F41.9	Anxiety disorder, unspecified
F42	**Obsessive-compulsive disorders**
F42.0	Predominantly obsessional thoughts or ruminations
F42.1	Predominantly compulsive acts (obsessional rituals)
F42.2	Mixed obsessional thoughts and acts
F42.8	Other obsessive-compulsive disorders
F42.9	Obsessive-compulsive disorder, unspecified
F43	**Reaction to severe stress, and adjustment disorders**
F43.0	Acute stress reaction
F43.1	Post-traumatic stress disorder

ICD-10 Classification of Anxiety and Stress-Related Disorders	
F43	**Reaction to severe stress, and adjustment disorders (cont.)**
F43.2	Adjustment disorders
F43.20	Brief depressive reaction
F43.21	Prolonged depressive reaction
F43.22	Mixed anxiety and depressive reaction
F43.23	With predominant disturbance of other emotions
F43.24	With predominant disturbance of conduct
F43.25	With mixed disturbance of emotions and conduct
F43.26	With other specified predominant symptoms
F43.8	Other reactions to severe stress
F43.9	Reaction to severe stress, unspecified

DSM-IV-TR Classification of Anxiety and Stress-Related Disorders	
Panic and anxiety disorders	
291.89	Alcohol-induced anxiety disorder
292.89	Substance-induced anxiety disorder (specify substance)
293.84	Anxiety disorder due to general medical condition
300.00	Anxiety disorder NOS
300.01	Panic disorder without agoraphobia
300.02	Generalized anxiety disorder (GAD)
300.21	Panic disorder with agoraphobia
Phobias	
300.22	Agoraphobia without history of panic disorder
300.23	Social phobia (specify if Generalized)
300.29	Specific phobia (specify type: animal/injection/blood/injury/situation/other)
Obsessive-compulsive disorders	
300.3	Obsessive-compulsive disorder (specify if with poor insight)
301.4	Obsessive-compulsive personality disorder (Axis II)
Adjustment disorders	
309.0	Adjustment disorder with depressed mood
309.24	Adjustment disorder with anxiety
309.28	Adjustment disorder with mixed anxiety and depressed mood
309.3	Adjustment disorder with disturbance of conduct
309.4	Adjustment disorder with mixed disturbance of emotions and conduct
309.9	Adjustment disorder unspecified

DSM-IV-TR Classification of Anxiety and Stress-Related Disorders	
Other stress-related disorders	
308.3	Acute stress disorder
309.21	Separation anxiety disorder
309.81	Post-traumatic stress disorder (specify if acute/chronic, with delayed onset)

3.3 Panic Disorder

Panic disorder is a syndrome characterized by recurrent unexpected panic attacks about which there is persistent concern.

3.3.1 Epidemiology

- In the general population, the prevalence of panic disorder is approximately 1%–4%
- Prevalence is higher in primary care or medical settings
- There is a bimodal distribution of incidence with one peak in late adolescence and another smaller peak in adulthood
- More commonly diagnosed in women (2:1 female/male ratio)

3.3.2 Etiology

Genetic Factors

The morbid risk for panic disorder in relatives of probands is 15%–30%, much higher than in the general population (2%). Female relatives are at higher risk than male relatives

Life Events

There is an excess of stressful life events in the year prior to onset of panic disorder, especially illness or death of cohabitants or close relatives

Physiological Factors

Abnormalities in cholinergic receptors

Dysregulation

Dysregulation of 5-HT, NE, CRF, glutamate, and GABA has been implicated

3.3.3   Symptoms

Panic attacks are discrete episodes of intense anxiety which develop abruptly and peak within 10 minutes. They are associated with at least 4 other symptoms of autonomic arousal including:

Cardiac Symptoms
- Palpitations
- Tachycardia
- Chest pain or discomfort

Gastro-Intestinal Symptoms
- Nausea
- Abdominal distress

Neurological Symptoms
- Trembling and shaking
- Dizziness
- Light-headedness
- Faintness
- Paresthesias

- Pulmonary symptoms
- Shortness of breath
- A feeling of choking

Autonomic Arousal
- Sweating
- Chills
- Hot flashes

Psychological Symptoms
- Derealization
- Depersonalization
- A fear of losing control
- A fear of dying

3.3.4   Diagnosis

Panic Disorder (episodic paroxysmal anxiety) (F41.0, 300.01/300.21)
Prototypical Symptoms per ICD-10
• Recurrent attacks of severe anxiety (panic) which are not restricted to any particular situation or set of circumstances, and which are therefore unpredictable • Sudden onset of palpitations, chest pain, choking sensations, dizziness, and feelings of unreality (depersonalization or derealization) • A secondary fear of dying, losing control, or going mad • Often followed by a persistent fear of having another attack
ICD-10 Diagnostic Guidelines
Several severe attacks of autonomic anxiety should have occurred within a period of about **1 month**: • In circumstances where there is no objective danger • Without being confined to known or predictable situations • With comparative freedom from anxiety symptoms between attacks (although anticipatory anxiety is common) Rule out phobias, medical conditions, substance abuse, or other anxiety disorders

Panic Disorder (episodic paroxysmal anxiety) (F41.0, 300.01/300.21)
Summary of DSM-IV-TR Diagnostic Guidelines
Repeated and sudden panic attacks, at least one of which is followed by persistent behavior-altering anxiety about further attacks and their consequences. **For exact diagnostic criteria, please refer to the DSM-IV-TR.**

DSM-IV-TR Diagnostic qualifiers	
• 300.01: Without agoraphobia	• 300.21: With agoraphobia

3.3.5 Differential Diagnosis

Psychiatric Conditions
- Anxiety due to a general medical condition
- Substance-induced anxiety disorder
- Other anxiety disorders
- Psychotic disorders
- Social phobia
- Specific phobia
- Generalized Anxiety Disorder (GAD)
- Obsessive-Compulsive Disorder (OCD)
- Post-Traumatic Stress Disorder (PTSD)
- Delusional disorder

Medical Conditions
- Hyperthyroidism
- Congestive heart failure
- Chronic obstructive pulmonary disease
- Myocardial infarction

3.3.6 Treatment

Psychotherapy
- CBT is a preferred and effective treatment for panic disorder
- Behavioral therapy and CBT are equally effective in reducing anxiety in panic disorder
- Panic focused CBT and exposure therapy

Pharmacotherapy
- Pharmacotherapy is an effective treatment for panic disorder
- SSRIs are recommended as the drugs of choice. Beneficial effect may take 3-8 weeks
- Alternative antidepressants include TCAs. Clomipramine has been shown to be 70%-80% effective

Pharmacotherapy (cont.)
- Benzodiazepines (alprazolam or clonazepam) should be used with caution due to potential for abuse/dependence/cognitive impairment. This is effective for severe, frequent, and incapacitating symptoms
- Venlafaxine is proving effective in clinical trials

Combination Therapy

The combination of CBT and pharmacotherapy is slightly more effective than CBT alone

3.3.7   Comorbidity

- 10%–65% of patients have at least one co-morbid psychiatric disorder.
- Common comorbid psychiatric conditions include the following:
  - Major depression (10%–65%)
  - Bipolar Disorder →101
  - Substance related disorder
  - Social phobia and Generalized Anxiety Disorder (GAD)
  - Specific phobia
  - Obsessive Compulsive Disorder (OCD)
  - Post Traumatic Stress Disorder (PTSD)
- Common comorbid medical conditions
  - COPD
  - Hyperthyroidism
  - Cardiac arrhythmias
  - Dizziness

3.4   Generalized Anxiety Disorder

Generalized Anxiety Disorder (GAD) is a chronic disabling psychiatric condition characterized by excessive anxiety and worry that is difficult to control.

3.4.1   Epidemiology

- Lifetime prevalence is approximately 5%–6%
- GAD is more common in females and younger individuals
- The average age at onset is between 15 and 25 years
- The female to male ratio is 4:3
- Incidence is approximately 3% each year
- GAD is the most common anxiety disorder diagnosed in the elderly

3.4.2   Etiology

- GABA, glutamate, monoamine and/or neuropeptide dysregulation
- Altered structure and function in brain regions implicated in emotion processing

3.4.3 Symptoms

The symptoms of anxiety include impaired concentration, restlessness, fatigue, irritability, muscle tension and sleep disturbances. GAD is distinguished from normal worrying in that its anxiety symptoms are higher in intensity, longer in duration, and significantly impair daily function.

Psychological Symptoms	Physiological Symptoms

• Uncontrollable worry
• Apprehension
• Fear
	• Increased muscle tension
	  - Trembling
	  - Headaches
	  - Neck or back pain
	• Increased autonomic hyperactivity
	  - Shortness of breath
	  - Sweating, clamminess
	  - Palpitations
	  - Dry mouth
	  - Diarrhea
	  - Nausea
	  - Frequent urination

3.4.4 Diagnosis

Generalized Anxiety Disorder (F41.1, 300.02)
Prototypical Symptoms per ICD-10
• Anxiety which is generalized and persistent but not restricted to, or even strongly predominating in, any particular environmental circumstances • Continuous feelings of nervousness, trembling, muscular tension, sweating, lightheadedness, palpitations, dizziness, and epigastric discomfort • Fears that the sufferer or a relative will shortly become ill or have an accident are often expressed, together with a variety of other worries and forebodings

Generalized Anxiety Disorder (F41.1, 300.02)

ICD-10 Diagnostic Criteria

The patient must have primary symptoms of anxiety on **most days for at least several weeks at a time**, and usually for several months. These symptoms should usually involve elements of:

- Apprehension (worries about future misfortunes, feeling "on edge", difficulty in concentrating, etc)
- Motor tension (restless fidgeting, tension headaches, trembling, inability to relax)
- Autonomic overactivity (lightheadedness, sweating, tachycardia or tachypnoea, epigastric discomfort, dizziness, dry mouth, etc)

Rule out depressive episode, phobic anxiety disorder, panic disorder, or obsessive-compulsive disorder

Summary of DSM-IV-TR Diagnostic Guidelines

Anxiety symptoms that are difficult to control occur **on most days for at least 6 months**, and cannot be attributed to other psychiatric disorders, medical conditions or substance abuse.

For exact diagnostic criteria, please refer to the DSM IV-TR.

3.4.5 Management

1. First assess medical and substance-related causes of anxiety symptoms
2. Medical workup includes:
   - Medical history
   - Psychiatric history
   - Family history of medical and psychiatric disorders
   - Physical examination
   - Neurological examination
   - Laboratory studies:
     - Electrolytes
     - CBC
     - Fasting blood glucose
     - Calcium level
     - TFT
     - LFT
     - Urine for drug screening (if suspected)
     - Special laboratory studies depending on symptomatology

3.4.6   Rating Scales

- Hamilton Anxiety Scale
- Self Rating Scales:
  - Beck Anxiety Inventory
  - State Trait Anxiety Inventory

3.4.7   Treatment

Nonpharmacologic Treatments (First line)

- Exercise
- Sleep hygiene
- Relaxation
- Cognitive behavioral therapy
- Individual and dynamic therapies

Pharmacologic Treatments (Second line)

- Benzodiazepine
- Buspirone
- SSRIs
- SNRIs
- Alpha-adrenergic antagonists

Cognitive Behavioral Therapy

Involves cognitive restructuring, exposure to worrying'1 thoughts and relaxation are recommended as a first line intervention

Combination Therapy

There is limited evidence for the efficacy of combined pharmacotherapy and psychotherapy in the treatment of GAD

3.4.8   Comorbid Conditions

- Major depressive disorder (MDD) (62%)
- Alcohol dependence (37%)
- Other anxiety disorders

3.5   Obsessive Compulsive Disorder

3.5.1   Definitions

Obsessions

Recurrent, persistent, intrusive ideas, thoughts, images, or impulses that the patient regards as alien and absurd, while recognizing them as products of his/her own mind. Attempts are made to ignore and suppress them.

Compulsions

Voluntary motor actions which are reluctantly performed despite being regarded as alien or absurd. The act is performed with a subjective sense of obsession coupled with a desire to resist it. When the individual does attempt to resist, there is a mounting sense of tension which can only be relieved by yielding. It is traditionally understood that patients with OCD are attempting to neutralize the anxiety caused by their obsessions by carrying out their compulsions.

3.5.2 Epidemiology

- Prevalence rate is approximately 2% worldwide
- Most cases of OCD begin prior to adulthood and approximately one third to one half of adult OCD cases have a childhood onset, with approximately 20% of cases starting by age 10
- The age of onset is bimodal between ages 6 and 15 for males and between ages 20 and 29 for females

3.5.3 Etiology

Genetics

- Up to 20% first degree relatives have subclinical OCD symptoms

Neurochemistry

- Dysregulation of the 5HT system and/or 5HT/DA systems are potentially involved in the development and expression of the disorder
- Abnormalities in the glutamate receptors

Neuroanatomy

- Abnormalities in the cortical-striatal-thalamo-cortical circuitry (CSTC)
- Basal ganglia abnormalities
- Dysregulation of limbic circuitry

Premorbid Personality

- The obsessive-compulsive personality disorder is associated with OCD

Psychoanalytic Theory

- Defensive regression to pregenital anal-erotic stage of development
- Defensive mechanism against aggressive and cruel impulses
- Key defenses: Reaction formation, isolation

3.5.4   Symptom Clusters of OCD

Symptom Clusters of OCD [6]			
Obsessions (%)		**Compulsions (%)**	
Contamination	45%	Checking	60%
Pathological doubt	42%	Washing	50%
Somatic	36%	Counting	35%
Need for symmetry	31%	Need to confess	31%
Aggressive impulse	28%	Symmetry/precision	28%
Sexual impulse	26%	Hoarding	18%
Other	13%	Multiple compulsions	48%
Multiple obsessions	60%		

3.5.5   Diagnosis

Obsessive-Compulsive Disorder (F42, 300.3)
Prototypical Symptoms per ICD-10
<ul><li>Recurrent obsessional thoughts (ideas, images or impulses that enter the individual's mind again and again in a stereotyped form) or compulsive acts (stereotyped behaviors that are repeated again and again, are not inherently enjoyable, nor do they result in the completion of inherently useful tasks)</li><li>Usually, though not invariably, this behavior is recognized by the individual as pointless or ineffectual and repeated attempts are made to resist it; in very long-standing cases, resistance may be minimal</li><li>Autonomic anxiety symptoms are often present, but distressing feelings of internal or psychic tension without obvious autonomic arousal are also common</li></ul>
ICD-10 Diagnostic Guidelines
Obsessional symptoms or compulsive acts, or both, must be present on **most days for at least 2 successive weeks** and be a source of distress or interference with activities. The obsessional symptoms should have the following characteristics:<ul><li>They must be recognized as the individual's own thoughts or impulses</li><li>There must be at least one thought or act that is still resisted unsuccessfully, even though others may be present which the sufferer no longer resists.</li><li>The thought of carrying out the act must not in itself be pleasurable (simple relief of tension or anxiety is not regarded as pleasure in this sense)</li><li>The thoughts, images, or impulses must be unpleasantly repetitive</li></ul>Obsessional symptoms developing in the presence of schizophrenia, Tourette's syndrome, or organic mental disorder should be regarded as part of these conditions.

Obsessive-Compulsive Disorder (F42, 300.3)

Summary of DSM-IV-TR Diagnostic Guidelines

OCD presents with obsessive or compulsive symptoms recognized by the patient to be excessive and unreasonable, that are time consuming and interfere with functioning, and that are not caused by substance abuse or general medical conditions.

For exact diagnostic criteria, please refer to the DSM-IV-TR.

3.5.6 Differential Diagnosis

- Tourette's/tic Disorders
- Obsessive Compulsive Personality Disorder (OCPD)
- OCD Spectrum Disorders
- Eating Disorders
- Psychotic Disorders
- Depressive Disorders
- Anxiety Disorders
- Pervasive Developmental Disorders (PDD)
- Delusional Disorder (typically somatic type)

3.5.7 Treatment

Psychotherapy

Cognitive behavioral therapy involving graded exposure to anxiety-provoking stimuli and ritualizing prevention is recommended as a first line intervention

Pharmacotherapy

- First line agents include SSRIs: Fluoxetine, sertraline, fluvoxamine, paroxetine, citalopram, and escitalopram
- TCAs: Clomipramine
- Augmentation of SSRIs with atypical antipsychotics in refractory cases. Maintenance therapy for at least 1-2 years. Relapse is common. Long term treatment indicated after two relapses

Combination Therapy

CBT with pharmacotherapy. The decision of combination therapy is based on the severity of the OCD and any co-morbid conditions that may benefit from pharmacotherapy

3.5.8 Comorbid Conditions

- OCPD and other Personality Disorders
- Major depression and other Mood Disorders
- Eating disorders
- Other anxiety disorders: Panic disorder, social phobia, specific phobia
- OCD spectrum disorders
- Tic disorders

3.5.9   Prognosis

- Many patients have a chronic waxing and waning course
- Approximately one third to one half of patients with a pediatric onset will have symptoms that continue to adulthood
- Approximately 15% of patients have progressive deterioration in occupational and social functioning

Poor Prognostic Factors

- Comorbid psychiatric disorder
- Earlier onset
- Longer duration of illness
- Poor insight into the illness
- More severe, bizarre symptoms; symmetry, ordering, hoarding obsessions
- Need for hospitalization because of severe symptoms

Good Prognostic Factors

- Obsessions without accompanying compulsions
- Presence of a precipitating event
- Episodic rather than chronic symptoms
- Overall good/social occupational adjustment

3.5.10   Workup for OCD

- Detailed history
- Collateral information
- Yale-Brown Obsessive Compulsive Scale (Y-BOCS)
  - 10-item severity rating scale: 0 = no symptoms to 40 = severe symptoms

3.6   Traumatic Stress Disorders

3.6.1   Temporal Criteria

Acute Stress Disorder

- Develops within 1 month and lasts for 2 days–4 weeks

Post-Traumatic Stress Disorder

- Duration more than 1 month
- Acute <3 months
- Chronic >3 months
- 6 months after stressor: Delayed onset

3.6.2   Post-Traumatic Stress Disorder (PTSD)

Epidemiology

- Lifetime risk of exposure to a trauma is approximately 39%
- Lifetime risk of developing PTSD is approximately 8%
- PTSD affects women more than men. Female to male ratio is 2:1. Females 10.4% and males 5%

Diagnosis

Post-Traumatic Stress Disorder (PTSD) (F43.1, 309.81)
Prototypical Symptoms per ICD-10
• Episodes of repeated reliving of the trauma in intrusive memories ("flashbacks") or dreams, occurring against the persisting background of a sense of "numbness" and emotional blunting, detachment from other people, unresponsiveness to surroundings, anhedonia, and avoidance of activities and situations reminiscent of the trauma
• Fear and avoidance of cues that remind the sufferer of the original trauma
• Usually a state of autonomic hyperarousal with hypervigilance, an enhanced startle reaction, and insomnia
• Anxiety and depression are commonly associated with the above symptoms
• and signs, and suicidal ideation is not infrequent; excessive use of alcohol or drugs may be a complicating factor
• Rarely, there may be dramatic, acute bursts of fear, panic or aggression, triggered by stimuli arousing a sudden recollection and/or re-enactment of the trauma or of the original reaction to it
ICD-10 Diagnostic Guidelines
• Evidence that the disorder arose within **6 months** of a traumatic event of an exceptionally threatening or catastrophic nature, which is likely to cause pervasive distress in almost anyone (eg, natural or man-made disaster, combat, serious accident, witnessing the violent death of others, or being the victim of torture, terrorism, rape, or other crime).
• A repetitive, intrusive recollection or re-enactment of the event in memories, daytime imagery, or dreams.

Post-Traumatic Stress Disorder (PTSD) (F43.1, 309.81)
Summary of DSM-IV-TR Diagnostic Guidelines

- Exposure to a traumatic event that threatened severe injury or death to self or others, and to which the response was immediate intense fear and helplessness, followed by persistent symptoms of reliving the event, hyperarousal, detachment and other psychological disturbances
- Presence of distressing symptoms that include reliving the traumatic event through intrusive thoughts, hyperarousal, avoidance of memories, event amnesia, and affective blunting

For exact diagnostic criteria, please refer to the DSM IV-TR.

Diagnostic Tools

- PTSD Checklist (self-reported scale)
- Impact of Events Scale (self-reported)
- Davidson Trauma Scale (self-reported)
- Clinician Administered PTSD Scale (structured interview)
- Structured interview for PTSD (structured diagnostic interview)
- Rates of PTSD are related to specific types of traumatic events (Ressler etc. 1995)
  - Rape: 65%
  - Combat: 38.8%
  - Natural disaster: 3.7%
  - Criminal assault: 1.8%

PTSD-Associated Features

- Depression
- Anger, isolation, social withdrawal
- Shame, survivors guilt
- Self-blame and self-harming behaviors
- History of multiple traumas
- Early physical, emotional and/or sexual abuse

Differential Diagnosis

- Acute stress disorder
- Personality disorders
- Major depressive disorder (MDD)
- Malingering/factitious disorder
- Substance use
- Adjustment disorder
- Bipolar disorder

Treatment

Psychotherapy

- Cognitive behavioral therapy with graded exposure to imagery
- Eye movement desensitization and reprocessing (EMDR) has been shown to have similar efficacy to CBT
- Psychodynamic psychotherapy may be used to explore the connection between the trauma and its effects
- Relaxation training
- Group therapy

Pharmacotherapy

- SSRIs are a first line treatment
- TCAs and MAOIs may also be useful
- Benzodiazepines for anxiety and insomnia (high risk of dependence and abuse potential)
- Atypical antipsychotics
- Antiadrenergics

Comorbidity

- 80% have another lifetime diagnosis
- Most common are MDD, alcohol abuse/dependence, social phobia and agoraphobia
- Other anxiety disorders

Prognosis

- 55% recover within nine months
- 15%-25% have a chronic course

Good Prognostic Factors

- Healthy premorbid function
- Brief trauma of lesser severity
- No personal or family history of psychiatric illness
- Good social support
- Absence of maladaptive coping mechanisms (avoidance, denial, not talking about the problems, thought suppression or rumination)

3.6.3   Acute Stress Disorder

Introduction

This disorder describes an acute response to trauma. It includes the criteria for PTSD but adds and emphasizes dissociative symptoms.

	PTSD	ASD
Intrusive Recollections	✓	✓
Avoidance of reminders of the trauma	✓	✓
Hyperarousal	✓	✓
Duration	> 1 month	< 1 month
Emphasis on Dissociative Symptoms	Less	More

Prevalence

Approximately 7% to 33% of trauma sufferers develop ASD, and 75% to 85% of people with ASD go on to develop PTSD.

Diagnosis

Acute Stress Reaction/Disorder (F43.0, 308.3)*
Prototypical Symptoms per ICD-10
• Symptoms show great variation but typically they include an initial state of "daze", with some constriction of the field of consciousness and narrowing of attention, inability to comprehend stimuli, and disorientation
• Initial state may be followed either by further withdrawal from the surrounding situation (to the extent of a dissociative stupor), or by agitation and over-activity (flight reaction or fugue)
• Autonomic signs of panic anxiety (tachycardia, sweating, flushing) are commonly present
• Partial or complete amnesia for the episode may be present
• The symptoms usually appear within minutes of the impact of the stressful stimulus or event, and disappear within 2-3 days (often within hours)

Acute Stress Reaction/Disorder (F43.0,308.3)*

ICD-10 Diagnostic Guidelines

There must be an immediate and clear temporal connection between the impact of an exceptional stressor and the onset of symptoms; onset is usually within a few minutes, if not immediate. In addition, the symptoms:

- Show a mixed and usually changing picture; in addition to the initial state of "daze", depression, anxiety, anger, despair, overactivity, and withdrawal may all be seen, but no one type of symptom predominates for long
- Resolve rapidly (within a few hours at the most) in those cases where removal from the stressful environment is possible; in cases where the stress continues or cannot by its nature be reversed, the symptoms **usually begin to diminish after 24–48 hours and are usually minimal after about 3 days**

Summary of DSM-IV-TR Diagnostic Guidelines

- Exposure to a traumatic event in which the person experienced, witnessed, or was confronted with an event that involved actual or threatened death or serious injury, or a threat to the physical integrity of self or others causing a response of intense fear, helplessness, or horror
- Symptoms include dissociative symptoms (eg, numbing, sense of detachment), re-experiencing of the event, avoidance of reminders, anxiety and increased arousal, hypervigilance, exaggerated startle response

For exact diagnostic criteria, please refer to the DSM-IV-TR.

*The ICD-10 categorizes this as Acute Stress Reaction, which has symptoms similar to the Acute Stress Disorder specified in the DSM-IV-TR, but of much shorter duration - typically of 48 hours and resolving in less than 3 days vs. the DSM's specification of a maximum of 4 weeks.

Differential Diagnosis

- Post traumatic stress disorder (PTSD)
- Personality disorders
- Major depressive disorder (MDD)
- Malingering/factitious disorder
- Substance use

Diagnostic Tools

- Acute Stress Disorder Interview - Structured interview
- Acute Stress Disorder Scale (ASDS) - Self-report measure

Treatment

Psychotherapy
- Cognitive behavioral therapy (CBT)
- Exposure therapy
- Eye movement desensitization and reprocessing (EMDR)

Pharmacological
- SSRIs: Some support for use
- Benzodiazepines: Can be used symptomatically for anxiety and insomnia

3.7   Phobias

3.7.1   Introduction

Phobias fall into 3 generally recognized categories:
- Specific phobias: Related to a specific panic trigger such as spiders, snakes, dogs, water, flying, or other specific objects or situations.
- Social phobia: Related to fear of other people or social situations, performance anxiety, fear of embarrassment or scrutiny; may be generalized (eg, social anxiety disorder), or specific (eg, triggered by specific social situation)
- Agoraphobia: Generalized fear of leaving home or a safe area

3.7.2   Epidemiology

- The lifetime prevalence of phobia is about 10% in the general population
- Specific phobia often begins in childhood or adolescence and many vary based on subtype
- Age of onset peaks in childhood and in the mid 20s
- Prevalence is usually higher in women versus men (2:1)
- Prevalence rates differ for specific phobic subtypes

3.7.3   Diagnosis

Agoraphobia

Agoraphobia (F40.00/F40.01, 300.21/300.22)
Prototypical Symptoms per ICD-10
• Fear of open spaces and of related aspects such as the presence of crowds and the difficulty of immediate easy escape to a safe place (usually home) • An interrelated and often overlapping cluster of phobias involving fears of leaving home • Fear of entering shops, crowds, and public places, or of travelling alone in trains, buses, or planes • Sufferers may become completely housebound, or terrified by the thought of collapsing and being left helpless in public • Depressive and obsessional symptoms and social phobias may also be present but do not dominate the clinical picture

Agoraphobia (F40.00/F40.01, 300.21/300.22)

ICD-10 Diagnostic Guidelines

All of the following criteria should be fulfilled for a definite diagnosis:

- The psychological or autonomic symptoms must be primarily manifestations of anxiety and not secondary to other symptoms, such as delusions or obsessional thoughts
- The anxiety must be restricted to (or occur mainly in) **at least 2 of the following situations:** Crowds, public places, travelling away from home, travelling alone
- Avoidance of the phobic situation must be, or have been, a prominent feature

Diagnostic qualifiers ICD-10

• **F40.00** - Without panic disorder	**F40.01** - With panic disorder

Summary of DSM-IV-TR Diagnostic Guidelines

Agoraphobia is characterized by a fear of leaving one's home, or familiar or "safe" environment caused by anxiety about entering environments or situations perceived to be difficult or embarrassing to escape (eg, wide-open spaces, crowds, bridges, uncontrollable social situations or public spaces such as shopping malls, airports). Typically, this is a complication of panic disorder, although it can occasionally develop on its own.

For exact diagnostic criteria, please refer to the DSM-IV-TR.

Social Phobia

Social Phobias (F40.1, 300.23)

Prototypical Symptoms per ICD-10

- Phobias centered around a fear of scrutiny by other people in comparatively small groups (as opposed to crowds), usually leading to avoidance of social situations
- Usually start in adolescence equally common in men and women
- May be discrete (ie, restricted to eating in public, to public speaking, or to encounters with the opposite sex) or diffuse, involving almost all social situations outside the family circle
- Usually associated with low self-esteem and fear of criticism
- May present with blushing, hand tremor, nausea, or urgency of micturition, or outright panic attacks
- Marked avoidance, in extreme cases resulting in almost complete social isolation

Social Phobias (F40.1, 300.23)

Diagnostic criteria ICD-10

All of the following criteria should be fulfilled for a definite diagnosis:

- The psychological, behavioral, or autonomic symptoms must be primarily manifestations of anxiety and not secondary to other symptoms such as delusions or obsessional thoughts
- The anxiety must be restricted to or predominate in particular social situations
- The phobic situation is avoided whenever possible

Summary of DSM-IV-TR Diagnostic Guidelines

- Excessive and persistent fear of certain social or performance situations (eg, speaking in front of a group of people)
- Recognition that fear is unreasonable, but inability to control it
- Avoidance of the stimulus or endurance in significant distress, leading to behavior that interferes with the person's normal functioning or routine
- Other disorders such as GAD or panic disorder, general medical conditions, or substance abuse should be ruled out

For exact diagnostic criteria please refer to the DSM IV-TR.

Specific Phobias

Specific (isolated) Phobias (F40.3, 300.29)

Prototypical Symptoms per ICD-10

- A panic reaction restricted to highly specific situations such as proximity to particular animals, heights, thunder, darkness, flying, closed spaces, urinating or defecating in public toilets, eating certain foods, dentistry, the sight of blood or injury, and the fear of exposure to specific diseases
- The seriousness of the resulting handicap depends on how easy it is for the sufferer to avoid the phobic situation

ICD-10 Diagnostic Criteria

All of the following should be fulfilled for a definite diagnosis:

- The psychological or autonomic symptoms must be primary manifestations of anxiety, and not secondary to other symptoms such as delusion or obsessional thought
- The anxiety must be restricted to the presence of the particular phobic object or situation
- The phobic situation is avoided whenever possible

Specific (isolated) Phobias (F40.3, 300.29)

Summary of DSM-IV-TR Diagnostic Guidelines

- **Excessive fear of specific objects or situations** (eg, heights, closed spaces, certain animals, etc) that provokes significant anxiety or panic on exposure to feared stimulus
- Recognition that the fear is unreasonable, but inability to control it
- Avoidance of the stimulus or endurance in significant distress, leading to behavior that interferes with the person's normal functioning or routine
- Other disorders such as GAD, OCD or panic disorders should be ruled out

For exact diagnostic criteria, please refer to the DSM IV-TR.

3.7.4   Treatment

Psychological Treatment

- CBT including exposure therapy
- Behavior therapy
  - Exposure
  - Systematic desensitization
  - Participant modeling

Pharmacological Treatment

  - Benzodiazepines
  - Propranolol

Combination Therapy

3.7.5   Prognosis

- Typically, very good; a majority of people with specific and social phobias improve significantly with appropriate psycho- and pharmacotherapy
- Poor treatment adherence and prematurely quitting treatment results in a poorer prognosis

List of references

[5]   Kessler et al 2005a, 2005b. Archives of General Psychiatry

[6]   Rasmussen and Tsuang, 1986

4   Eating Disorders

4.1   Introduction

Eating disorders are characterized by disordered patterns of eating, accompanied by distress, disparagement, preoccupation and/or distraction associated with one's eating, weight, or body shape.

4.2   Classification

Classification of Eating Disorders	
ICD-10 Classification	
F50.0	Anorexia nervosa
F50.1	Atypical anorexia nervosa
F50.2	Bulimia nervosa
F50.3	Atypical bulimia nervosa
F50.4	Overeating associated with other psychological disturbances
F50.5	Vomiting associated with other psychological disturbances
F50.8	Other eating disorders
F50.9	Eating disorder, unspecified
DSM-IV-TR Classification	
307.1	Anorexia nervosa[1]
307.50	Eating disorder NOS
307.51	Bulimia nervosa[2]
307.52	Pica
307.53	Rumination disorder
307.59	Feeding disorder of infancy and early childhood
[1]Specify Restricting or Binge/Purging type [2]Specify Purging or Nonpurging type	

4.3   Anorexia Nervosa

4.3.1   Epidemiology

- Prevalence: 0.3%–1% of young adult females
- Male to female ratio: 1:10
- Onset: 15–19 years
- Occupation: High rates in ballet dancers, gymnasts
- Social class: Overrepresented in higher social classes

4.3.2   Etiology

- Psychological factors: Anxiety, difficulties with emotion regulation, disturbed body image, eating problems in early life, negative self-evaluation
- Familial factors: Enmeshment and overprotection, a dominant intrusive mother, a passive ineffectual father, rigid family structure with conflict avoidance, weak generational boundaries
- Cultural factors: The western "thinness conscious" culture, role conflict changing expectations for and by women, food as a form of communication
- Biological factors: Genetic predisposition, disturbance in serotonergic function
- Temperament factors

4.3.3   Diagnosis

Anorexia Nervosa (F50.0, 307.1)
Prototypical Symptoms per ICD-10
• Deliberate weight loss, induced and/or sustained by the patient
• Undernutrition of varying severity, with resulting secondary endocrine and metabolic changes and disturbances of bodily function

Anorexia Nervosa (F50.0, 307.1)

ICD-10 Diagnostic Guidelines

For a definite diagnosis, **all the following are required:**

- **Body weight is maintained at least 15% below that expected** (either lost or never achieved), or Quetelet's body-mass index is 17.5 or less (use if age >16 years). Prepubertal patients may show failure to make the expected weight gain during the period of growth
- The weight loss is self-induced by avoidance of "fattening foods". One or more of the following may also be present: self-induced vomiting; self-induced purging; excessive exercise; use of appetite suppressants and/or diuretics
- There is body-image distortion in the form of a specific psychopathology whereby a dread of fatness persists as an intrusive, overvalued idea and the patient imposes a low weight threshold on himself or herself
- A widespread endocrine disorder involving the hypothalamic-pituitary-gonadal axis is manifest in women as amenorrhea and in men as a loss of sexual interest and potency. (An apparent exception is the persistence of vaginal bleeds in anorexic women who are receiving replacement hormonal therapy, most commonly taken as a contraceptive pill.) There may also be elevated levels of growth hormone, raised levels of cortisol, changes in the peripheral metabolism of the thyroid hormone, and abnormalities of insulin secretion
- If onset is prepubertal, the sequence of pubertal events is delayed or even arrested (growth ceases; in girls the breasts do not develop and there is a primary amenorrhea; in boys the genitals remain juvenile). With recovery, puberty is often completed normally, but the menarche is late

Summary of DSM-IV-TR Diagnostic Guidelines

- Refusal to maintain body weight at or above a minimally normal weight for age and height (**<85% of expected**)
- Intense fear of gaining weight or becoming fat, even though underweight
- Disturbance in body weight and shape self-image, or denial of seriousness of low body weight
- Amenorrhea in postmenarcheal females

For exact diagnostic criteria, please refer to the DSM-IV-TR.

DSM-IV-TR Diagnostic Subtypes

- **Restricting Type:** Low body weight is maintained by dieting, excessive exercise or fasting, but no regular binging and/or purging
- **Binge eating/Purging Type:** Low weight maintained through binge eating and/or purging behavior, self-induced vomiting, or misuse of laxatives, diuretics or enemas

4.3.4   Differential Diagnosis

- GI disorders
- Endocrine disorders
- Occult malignancies
- Chronic infections
- Substance related disorders
- Other psychiatric disorders

4.3.5   Physiological Effects of Starvation in Anorexia Nervosa

- Cardiovascular: Bradycardia, hypotension, dysrhythmias, cardiac failure
- GI symptoms: Absent bowel sounds
- Dermatologic: Xerosis (dry, scaly skin), brittle hair and hair loss
- Endocrine and metabolic: Marked weight loss, emaciation, malnutrition, dehydration, electrolyte abnormalities, swollen parotids (from vomiting)
- Reproductive: Loss of libido, sterility, impotence
- Neurological: Seizures
- Hematologic: Blood count abnormalities, anemia
- Musculoskeletal: Muscle atrophy, weakness, low bone density

4.3.6   Criteria For Admission To Hospital

- Extremely low body weight: Less than 70% of ideal body weight
- Acute medical need:
  - Rapid, excessive weight loss
  - Unstable vital signs, bradycardia < 30 bpm or < 40 bpm with dizziness, hypothermia (core temp < 35°C/95°F)
  - Cardiac dysrhythmias other than sinus bradycardia
  - Marked dehydration, malnutrition signs (eg, cardiac failure, liver failure, pancreatitis, syncope, seizures, electrolyte disturbances)
  - Psychosis or significant risk of suicide
  - Other serious psychiatric comorbidities
  - Failure of outpatient treatment

4.3.7   Prognosis

- Approximately 45%-60% recover over 5-10 years
- 20%-30% continue to have residual moderate symptoms
- 10%-20% remain chronically ill
- Anorexia nervosa has a high mortality rate of 5%
- Women with anorexia nervosa are 12 times more likely to die than women in the general population
- The causes of death are medical complications (54%) and suicide (27%)

Poor Prognosis Factors
- Late age of onset
- Chronicity of illness > 6 years
- Lower initial minimum weight
- Bulimic features
- Obsessive compulsive personality features
- Male gender

4.3.8   Management

- Weight restoration and psychotherapy are the main treatments
- Medical evaluation
- Nutritional assessment and counseling
- Pharmacologic treatment

Medical Treatment	Nutritional Counseling	Psychiatric Treatment
• Antidepressants • Antipsychotics and mood stabilizers may help some anorexic patients when given as part of a complete treatment program	• Dietary patterns • Weight monitoring • Caloric requirements • Correcting nutritional/behavioral deficits	• Cognitive behavioral therapy (CBT) • Interpersonal psychotherapy (IPT) • Pharmacotherapy • Family therapy • Group psychotherapy

4.4   Bulimia Nervosa

4.4.1   Epidemiology

- 1% of young adult females
- 0.1% of men
- Peak onset is later than anorexia nervosa - late adolescence or early 20s
- BN is more common than AN
- About 30% of BN cases have a prior history of AN

4.4.2   Etiology

- Individual factors: Mood swings, chronic anxiety, poor impulse control, difficulty expressing anger, poor self-esteem
- Family factors: Volatile and conflicted family atmosphere, family history of depressive disorder, substance use, unreasonable high expectations, verbal, physical or sexual abuse
- Societal factors: Idealization of thinness, excessive focus on self-appearance, equate overweight with lack in self-control
- Biological factors: Dysregulation of eating related to serotonergic and dopaminergic mechanism

4.4.3   Diagnosis

Bulimia Nervosa (F50.2, 307.51)

Prototypical Symptoms per ICD-10

- Repeated bouts of overeating and an excessive preoccupation with the control of body weight, leading the patient to adopt extreme measures so as to mitigate the "fattening" effects of ingested food
- Repeated vomiting is likely to give rise to disturbances of body electrolytes, physical complications (tetany, epileptic seizures, cardiac arrhythmias, muscular weakness), and further severe loss of weight

ICD-10 Diagnostic Guidelines

For a definite diagnosis, **all the following are required:**

- A persistent preoccupation with eating, and an irresistible craving for food; the patient succumbs to episodes of overeating in which large amounts of food are consumed in short periods of time
- The patient attempts to counteract the "fattening" effects of food by one or more of the following: self-induced vomiting; purgative abuse, alternating periods of starvation; use of drugs such as appetite suppressants, thyroid preparations or diuretics. When bulimia occurs in diabetic patients they may choose to neglect their insulin treatment
- A morbid dread of fatness causing the patient to set herself or himself a sharply defined weight threshold, well below the premorbid weight that constitutes the optimum or healthy weight in the opinion of the physician

Summary of DSM-IV-TR Diagnostic Guidelines

- Recurrent episodes of binge eating characterized by eating in a discrete period of time an amount of food that is definitely larger than most people would eat during a similar period of time and under similar circumstances accompanied by a sense of lack of control over eating during the episode
- Engaging in recurrent inappropriate compensatory behavior in order to prevent weight gain (eg, vomiting, laxatives, diuretics, enemas, fasting, excessive exercise)
- Body shape and weight play exaggerated role in self-image
- Binge-purge episodes do not occur exclusively during episodes of Anorexia Nervosa

For exact diagnostic criteria, please refer to the DSM-IV-TR.

Diagnostic subtypes DSM-IV

- **Purging Type:** Engagement in purging behavior (eg, self-induced vomiting or the misuse of laxatives, diuretics, or enemas)
- **Non-Purging Type:** Engagement in other inappropriate compensatory behavior (eg, fasting or excessive exercise), but not purging behavior

4.4.4   Differential Diagnosis

- Gastro-intestinal disorders
- Occult malignancies
- Intestinal infection
- Connective tissue disorders
- Substance related disorders
- Other psychiatric disorders

4.4.5   Treatment

- Assessment: Medical evaluation, psychiatric evaluation
- Outpatient management is typical
- Nutritional counseling
- Psychotherapy: CBT, IPT
- Pharmacotherapy

4.4.6   Comorbidity

- Anxiety disorders (especially social phobia)
- Depressive disorder
- Substance abuse disorders
- Personality disorders

4.5   Binge Eating Disorder (BED)

Proposed DSM-V Diagnostic Criteria for Binge Eating Disorder*

- Recurrent episodes of binge eating. An episode of binge eating is characterized by both eating, in a discrete period of time an amount of food that is definitely larger than most people would eat in a similar period of time under similar circumstances, and a sense of lack of control over eating during the episode
- The binge-eating episodes are associated with 3 (or more) of the following:
  - Eating much more rapidly than normal
  - Eating until feeling uncomfortably full
  - Eating large amounts of food when not feeling physically hungry
  - Eating alone because of feeling embarrassed by how much one is eating
  - Feeling disgusted with oneself, depressed, or very guilty after overeating
- Marked distress regarding binge eating is present
- The binge eating is not associated with the recurrent use of inappropriate compensatory behavior and does not occur exclusively during the course Bulimia Nervosa or Anorexia Nervosa

*Not currently classified as a separate eating disorder in either the ICD-10 or the DSM-IV-TR.

5 Mood Disorders

5.1 Classification

ICD-10 Classification of Mood Disorders	
F30	**Manic episode**
F30.0	Hypomania
F30.1	Mania without psychotic symptoms
F30.2	Mania with psychotic symptoms
F30.8	Other manic episodes
F30.9	Manic episode, unspecified
F31	**Bipolar affective disorder**
F31.0	Current episode hypomanic
F31.1	Current episode manic without psychotic symptoms
F31.2	Current episode manic with psychotic symptoms
F31.3	Current episode mild or moderate depression
F31.30	Without somatic syndrome
F31.31	With somatic syndrome
F31.4	Current episode severe depression without psychotic symptoms
F31.5	Current episode severe depression with psychotic symptoms
F31.6	Current episode mixed
F31.7	Currently in remission
F31.8	Other bipolar affective disorders
F31.9	Bipolar affective disorder, unspecified
F32	**Depressive episode**
F32.0	Mild depressive episode
F32.00	Without somatic syndrome
F32.01	With somatic syndrome
F32.1	Moderate depressive episode
F32.10	Without somatic syndrome
F32.11	With somatic syndrome
F32.2	Severe depressive episode without psychotic symptoms
F32.3	Severe depressive episode with psychotic symptoms
F32.8	Other depressive episodes
F32.9	Depressive episode, unspecified

ICD-10 Classification of Mood Disorders	
F33	**Recurrent depressive disorder**
F33.0	Current episode mild
F33.00	Without somatic syndrome
F33.01	With somatic syndrome
F33.1	Current episode moderate
F33.10	Without somatic syndrome
F33.11	With somatic syndrome
F33.2	Current episode severe without psychotic symptoms
F33.3	Current episode severe with psychotic symptoms
F33.4	Currently in remission
F33.8	Other recurrent depressive disorders
F33.9	Recurrent depressive disorder, unspecified
F34	**Persistent mood (affective) disorders**
F34.0	Cyclothymia
F34.1	Dysthymia
F34.8	Other persistent mood (affective) disorders
F34.9	Persistent mood (affective) disorder, unspecified
F38	**Other mood (affective) disorders**
F38.0	Other single mood (affective) disorders
F38.00	Mixed affective episode
F38.1	Other recurrent mood (affective) disorders
F38.10	Recurrent brief depressive disorder
F38.8	Other specified mood (affective) disorders
F39	**Unspecified mood (affective) disorder**

DSM-IV-TR Classification of Mood Disorders	
Bipolar I disorder*	
296.0x	Single Manic Episode
296.40	Most Recent Episode Hypomanic
296.4x	Most Recent Episode Manic
296.5x	Most Recent Episode Depressed
296.6x	Most Recent Episode Mixed
296.7	Most Recent Episode Unspecified
Major depressive disorder (MDD)*	
296.2x	Single Episode
296.3x	Recurrent

DSM-IV-TR Classification of Mood Disorders	
Other mood disorders or features	
290.43	Vascular Dementia, With Depressed Mood
291.89	Alcohol-Induced Mood Disorder
292.84	Substance-Induced Mood Disorder
293.83	Mood Disorder due to General Medical Condition
296.80	Bipolar Disorder NOS
296.89	Bipolar II Disorder[1]
296.90	Mood Disorder NOS
300.4	Dysthymic Disorder[2]
301.13	Cyclothymic Disorder
309.0	Adjustment Disorder With Depressed Mood
309.28	Adjustment Disorder With Mixed Anxiety and Depressed Mood
311	Depressive Disorder NOS
*Current State Specifiers for Bipolar I and Major Depressive Disorder	
296.x1	Mild
296.x2	Single Episode, Moderate
296.x3	Severe Without Psychotic Features
296.x4	Severe With Psychotic Features (specify mood-congruent/incongruent)
296.x5	In Partial Remission
296.x6	In Full Remission

[1]Specify current/most recent episode hypomanic/depressed
[2]Specify if Early/Late Onset and if With Atypical Features

5.2   Unipolar Depressive Disorders

The DSM-IV denotes six categories of unipolar depressive disorders based on the number, duration and etiology (if known) of the depressive symptoms:
- Major depressive disorder (MDD)
- Dysthymic disorder
- Substance-induced mood disorder
- Mood disorder due to a general medical condition with depressive features
- Adjustment disorder with depressed mood
- Depressive disorder not otherwise specified (NOS)

5.3   Major Depressive Disorder (MDD)

5.3.1   Epidemiology

- Life time prevalence for MDD
  - Males 5%-12%
  - Females 10%-25%
- Point Prevalence
  - Males 2%-3%
  - Females 5%-9%

5.3.2   Risk Factors

- Genetic predisposition
- Negative childhood experiences (eg, child abuse)
- Predisposing personality traits (eg, melancholic, dependent)
- Psychosocial stressors:
  - Breakup of intimate relationship (eg, divorce, separation)
  - Economic hardship
  - Isolation
  - Complicated or prolonged bereavement
  - Specific stressors (eg, career, family, elderly care)
- Medical illness: Direct primary effect (eg, hypothyroidism) or secondary effect (eg, psychological response to poor health or serious illness such as cancer)
- Age: Age by itself does not appear to directly affect the rates of depression. Those over the age of 80 years do have higher rates, but this increase is primarily associated with medical illness, loss of function and independence, frailty, isolation, and other quality of life factors; well-functioning elderly adults do not experience this increase
- Drug side effect: Interferon, corticosteroids, beta-blockers
- Psychological factors. Based on **Beck's theory**, three concepts seek to explain the psychological substrate of depression:

Beck's cognitive triad
- A negative personal view
- A tendency to interpret his or her ongoing experience in a negative way
- A negative view of the future

Schemas
- Stable cognitive patterns forming the basis for the interpretation of situations

Cognitive distortions
- Systematic errors in thinking that maintain depressed people's beliefs in negative concepts

5.3.3   Diagnosis

MDD is diagnosed when a person has experienced at least one major depressive episode (MDE), but no manic, hypomanic or mixed episodes.

In general, the symptoms of depression can be remembered using the mnemonic **SIG E CAPS**:
- **S**leep: Increased or decreased sleep
- **I**nterest: Loss of interest in previously enjoyable activities
- **G**uilt: Increased feelings of guilt
- **E**nergy: Low energy, fatigue
- **C**oncentration: Decreased concentration
- **A**ppetite: Increased or decreased appetite
- **P**sychomotor: Psychomotor agitation or retardation
- **S**uicide: Suicidal ideation, plan, intent or recent or past attempt

These symptoms should not be explained by normal bereavement, substance abuse, general medical conditions, or other psychiatric disorders (eg, schizophrenia), and should cause significant distress and impairment of functioning. Specific ICD-10 and DSM-IV diagnostic criteria for depressive episodes and disorders are listed below.

ICD-10 Diagnostic Guidelines for Depressive Episodes (F32)	
Prototypical Symptoms and Features per ICD-10	
a.	Depressed mood, loss of interest and enjoyment, and reduced energy leading to increased fatigability and diminished activity
b.	Other **common symptoms:** • Marked tiredness after only slight effort • Reduced concentration and attention • Reduced self-esteem and self-confidence • Ideas of guilt and unworthiness • Bleak and pessimistic views of the future • Ideas or acts of self-harm or suicide • Disturbed sleep • Diminished appetite

ICD-10 Diagnostic Guidelines for Depressive Episodes (F32)
c.	Additional features:
	• Anxiety, distress, and motor agitation may be more prominent at times than the depression
	• Irritability, excessive consumption of alcohol, histrionic behavior, exacerbation of pre-existing phobic or obsessional symptoms, hypochondriacal preoccupations
	• Disruption in social or occupational activities, particularly for severe episodes
	• Atypical presentations are particularly common in adolescents
d.	Differentiation between mild, moderate, and severe depressive episodes rests upon a complicated clinical judgment that involves the number, type, and severity of symptoms present
e.	• **Single (first) depressive episodes** should be classified under single Depressive Episodes (**F32.x**) according to their intensity and features
	• **Repeated depressive episodes** should be classified as Recurrent Depressive Disorders (**F33.x**) according to their intensity and features

Somatic Symptoms of Depressive Episodes

For mild and moderate depressive episodes "**with somatic syndrome**" should be indicated if **at least 4 of the following symptoms** are present:

- Loss of interest or pleasure in activities that are normally enjoyable
- Lack of emotional reactivity to normally pleasurable surroundings and events
- Waking in the morning 2 hours or more before the usual time
- Depression worse in the morning
- Objective evidence of definite psychomotor retardation or agitation (remarked on or reported by other people)
- Marked loss of appetite
- Weight loss (often defined as 5% or more of body weight in the past month)
- Marked loss of libido

Mild Depressive Episode (F32.0)

- **At least 2 symptoms** of depressed mood, loss of enjoyment, or increased fatigability **plus at least 2 common symptoms** for **at least 2 weeks.**
- None of the symptoms should be present to an intense degree
- Some difficulty in continuing with ordinary work and social activities may be present
- Specify with (**F32.00**) or without (**F32.01**) somatic syndrome

ICD-10 Diagnostic Guidelines for Depressive Episodes (F32)

Moderate Depressive Episode (F32.1)

- **At least 2 symptoms** of depressed mood, loss of enjoyment, and increased fatigability **plus at least 3–4 common symptoms** for **at least 2 weeks.**
- Several symptoms are likely to be present to a marked degree
- Considerable difficulty in continuing with social, work or domestic activities likely present
- Specify with (**F32.10**) or without (**F32.11**) somatic syndrome

Severe depressive episode without psychotic symptoms (F32.2)

- **All 3 symptoms** of depressed mood, loss of enjoyment, and increased fatigability **plus at least 4 common symptoms** for **at least 2 weeks** (may make diagnosis sooner if symptoms are particularly severe)
- Considerable or severe distress, agitation, or retardation
- High risk of suicidality
- Significant or total impairment of social, work, or domestic activities

Severe depressive episode with psychotic symptoms (F32.3)

- **All 3 symptoms** of depressed mood, loss of enjoyment, and increased fatigability **plus at least 4 common symptoms** for **at least 2 weeks** (may make diagnosis sooner if symptoms are particularly severe)
- Presence of **delusions, hallucinations or depressive stupor**
  - Delusions usually involve ideas of sin, poverty, or imminent disasters
  - Auditory or olfactory hallucinations are usually of defamatory or accusatory voices or of rotting filth or decomposing flesh
  - Severe psychomotor retardation may progress to stupor
  - If required, delusions or hallucinations may be specified as mood-congruent or mood-incongruent
- Severe distress, agitation or retardation
- High risk of suicidality
- Significant or total impairment of social, work, or domestic activities

Other depressive episodes (F32.8)

- Episodes that do not fit depressive episodes described in F32.0–F32.3, but for which the overall diagnostic impression indicates that they are depressive in nature
- Examples include fluctuating mixtures of depressive symptoms (particularly the somatic variety) with nondiagnostic symptoms such as tension, worry, and distress, and mixtures of somatic depressive symptoms with persistent pain or fatigue not due to organic causes

ICD-10 Diagnostic Guidelines for Recurrent Depressive Disorder (F33)

Prototypical Symptoms and Features of Recurrent Depressive Disorders

- Repeated episodes of depression (mild, moderate or severe)
- No history of independent episodes of mood elevation and overactivity that fulfill the criteria of mania

Recurrent Depressive Disorder, Current Episode Mild (F33.0)

- Current episode fulfils the criteria for depressive episode, mild severity (F32.0)
- **At least 2 episodes** should have lasted a **minimum of 2 weeks** and should have been separated by several months without significant mood disturbance
- Indicate with (**F32.00**) or without (**F32.01**) somatic syndrome

Recurrent Depressive Disorder, Current Episode Moderate (F33.1)

- Current episode fulfils the criteria for depressive episode, moderate severity (F32.1)
- **At least 2 episodes** should have lasted a **minimum of 2 weeks** and should have been separated by several months without significant mood disturbance
- Indicate with (**F32.10**) or without (**F32.11**) somatic syndrome

Recurrent Depressive Disorder, Current Episode Severe Without Psychotic Features (F33.2)

- Current episode fulfils the criteria for depressive episode, severe without psychotic features (F32.2)
- **At least 2 episodes** should have lasted a **minimum of 2 weeks** and should have been separated by several months without significant mood disturbance

Recurrent Depressive Disorder, Current Episode Severe With Psychotic Features (F33.3)

- Current episode fulfils the criteria for depressive episode, severe with psychotic features (F32.3)
- **At least 2 episodes** should have lasted a **minimum of 2 weeks** and should have been separated by several months without significant mood disturbance

Recurrent Depressive Disorder, Currently in Remission (F33.4)

- The criteria for recurrent depressive disorder (F33.x) should have been fulfilled in the past, but the current state should not fulfill the criteria for depressive episode of any degree of severity or for any other disorder in F30-F39
- At least two episodes should have lasted a minimum of 2 weeks and should have been separated by several months without significant mood disturbance
- Otherwise the diagnosis should be other recurrent mood [affective] disorder (F38.1)
- This category can still be used if the patient is receiving treatment to reduce the risk of further episodes

Summary of DSM-IV-TR Diagnostic Guidelines for Major Depressive Episode and Disorder

Major Depressive Episode (296.2x, 296.3x, 296.5x)

- Depressed mood or loss of interest or pleasure in almost all activities plus presence of depressive symptoms
- Depressive symptoms include abrupt weight changes, insomnia/hypersomnia, psychomotor agitation/retardation, fatigue or low energy, feelings or worthlessness or guilt, diminished concentration, indecisiveness, suicidal ideation
- The symptoms do not meet criteria for mixed episode, and are not caused by bereavement, use of a substance, or a general medical condition
- The symptoms cause clinically significant distress and functional impairment

For exact diagnostic criteria, please refer to the DMS–IV-TR.

Severity Specifiers (code in 5th digit)

.x1	Mild
.x2	Moderate
.x3	Severe without psychotic features

.x4	Severe with psychotic features
	   - **Mood-congruent:** Psychosis along depressive themes
	   - **Mood-incongruent:** Persecutory delusions, thought insertion/broadcasting

.x5	In partial remission
.x6	In full remission
.x0	Unspecified

Qualitative Specifiers for Major Depressive Episodes*

Chronic	Full criteria for a major depressive episode have been met continuously for at least 2 years
With catatonic features	• Catalepsy or stupor • Excessive purposeless motor activity • Extreme negativism or mutism • Bizarre posturing, stereotyped movements, prominent mannerisms/grimacing • Echolalia or echopraxia
With melancholic features	• Loss of pleasure in activities • No reaction to pleasurable stimuli • Depressed mood • Depression regularly worse in the morning • Early morning awakening (>2 hours before usual time) • Psychomotor retardation or agitation • Significant anorexia or weight loss • Excessive or inappropriate guilt

Summary of DSM-IV-TR Diagnostic Guidelines for Major Depressive Episode and Disorder	
With atypical features	• Mood reactivity • Significant weight gain or increase in appetite • Hypersomnia • Leaden paralysis • Interpersonal rejection sensitivity
Postpartum onset	Onset of episode postpartum
With full interepisode recovery	Full remission is attained between the two most recent mood episodes
Without full interepisode recovery	Full remission is not attained between the two most recent mood episodes
With seasonal pattern	Temporal relationship between time of year and onset
*For exact specifier criteria, please refer to the DSM-IV-TR.	
Recurrent Major Depressive Episode, Major Depressive Disorder (MDD) (296.3x)	
• Repeated major depressive episodes more than 2 months apart • Not better accounted by mental disorders • No history of manic, mixed or hypomanic episodes **For exact diagnostic criteria, please refer to the DSM-IV-TR.**	

5.3.4   Differential Diagnosis of MDD

Many psychiatric, medical and pharmacological causes share some of the clinical features of MDD.

Psychiatric Conditions

- Mood disorders due to a general medical condition with depressive or with major depressive-like episode
- Dysthymic disorder
- Substance induced mood disorder with depressive features
- Dementia
- Bipolar disorder
- Attention deficit hyperactivity disorder
- Adjustment disorder with depressed mood
- Schizophrenia with negative symptoms

General Medical Conditions

- Cardiac disorders
- Respiratory disorders
- Endocrine disorders
- Infectious or inflammatory conditions
- Malignancy
- Metabolic deficiencies
- Nutritional deficiencies

Pharmacological Causes

- Analgesics
- Antibacterial agents
- Antineoplastic agents
- Cardiac and antihypertensive agents (eg, beta-blockers)
- Antipsychotic agents →206
- Anti-inflammatory agents (eg, corticosteroids)

5.3.5 Rating Scales

Montgomery–Asberg Depression Rating Scale (MADRS)					
		0 Points	2 Points	4 Points	6 Points
1	**Apparent Sadness:** Despondency, gloom, despair - reflected in speech, facial expression, posture. Rate by depth and inability to brighten up	No sadness	Looks dispirited but does brighten up without difficulty	Appears sad and unhappy most of the time	Looks miserable all the time. Extremely despondent
2	**Reported Sadness:** Reports of depressed mood, regardless if reflected in appearance or not. Includes low spirits, despondency or feeling of being beyond help and without hope	Occasional sadness in keeping with circumstances	Sad or low but brightens up without difficulty	Pervasive feelings of sadness or gloominess, influenced by external circumstances	Continuous or unvarying sadness, misery or despondency

MADRS (cont.)	0 Points	2 Points	4 Points	6 Points
3 **Inner Tension:** Feelings of edginess, mental tension mounting to panic, dread or anguish. Rate by intensity, frequency, duration, and extent of reassurance	Placid. Only fleeting inner tension	Occasional feelings of edginess and ill-defined discomfort	Continuous feelings of inner tension or intermittent panic	Unrelenting dread or anguish. Overwhelming panic
4 **Reduced Sleep:** Experience of reduced duration or depth of sleep compared with subject's normal pattern when well	Sleeps as normal	Difficulty dropping off or slightly reduced, light or fitful sleep	Moderate stiffness and resistance	Sleep reduced or broken by at least 2 hours
5 **Reduced Appetite:** Feeling of a loss of appetite. Rate by loss of desire for food or need to force oneself to eat	Normal or increased appetite	Slightly reduced appetite	No appetite. Food is tasteless	Needs persuasion to eat at all
6 **Concentration Difficulties:** In collecting one's thoughts. Rate by intensity, frequency, and degree of incapacity produced	No difficulties in concentrating	Occasional difficulties in collecting thoughts	Difficulties in concentrating, reduced ability to read or converse	Unable to read or converse without great difficulty
7 **Lassitude:** Difficulty in getting started or slowness in initiating and performing usual activities	Hardly any difficulty in getting started	Difficulties in starting activities	Difficulties in starting simple routine activities	Complete lassitude. Unable to do anything without help

MADRS (cont.)	0 Points	2 Points	4 Points	6 Points
8 **Inability to Feel:** Subjective experience of reduced interest in surroundings or activities. Reduced ability to react with adequate emotion to circumstances or people	Normal interest in the surroundings and in other people	Reduced ability to enjoy usual interests	Loss of interest in surroundings. Loss of feelings for friends	Experience of being emotionally paralyzed, inability to feel anger, grief, pleasure; complete failure to feel
9 **Pessimistic Thoughts:** Thoughts of guilt, inferiority, self-reproach, sinfulness, remorse, and ruin	No pessimistic thoughts	Fluctuating ideas of failure, self-reproach or self-depreciation	Persistent self-accusations, or definite, rational ideas of guilt or sin. Increasingly pessimistic	Delusions of ruin, remorse or irredeemable sin. Absurd, unshakable self-accusations
10 **Suicidal Thoughts:** Feeling life is not worth living, that a natural death would be welcome, suicidal thoughts, and preparations for suicide	Enjoys life or takes it as it comes	Weary of life. Only fleeting suicidal thoughts	Common, suicide considered as possible solution; without specific plans or intention	Explicit plans for suicide when there is an opportunity. Active preparations for suicide

MAD Rating Scale = points for all 10 parameters; **Minimum score**: 0, **maximum score**: 60

5.3.6   Management

- Ensure safety of patient: Assess suicidality, necessity for admission
- Consider nonpsychiatric differential diagnoses (eg, medical or drug causes), and attempt to clarify psychiatric diagnosis
- Collateral history from other source to verify information
- Special investigations to rule out other possible secondary causes of depression (CBC, UE, LFT, TFT, Ca, PO_4, Glucose, B12, Folate)
- Combined treatment approaches that include pharmacologic agents and psychotherapy have been found to be most effective

Treatment Approaches

Biological Agents
- SSRIs
- SNRIs
- Tricyclics
- Heterocyclics

Psychological Treatment
- Cognitive behavioral therapy
- Interpersonal therapy
- Combination of psychotherapy and antidepressants

Self-Management of Depression
- Physical exercise
- Bibliotherapy
- Computerized psychotherapy
- Increasing peer support

Treatment Phases
- The acute phase (up to 12 weeks, to achieve full remission)
- The continuation phase (lasts from 4 to 6 months)
- The maintenance phase (long term commitment to prophylactic treatment with an antidepressant)

5.3.7 Co-morbid Features of Depression

About two thirds of patients will also meet criteria for another psychiatric disorder:
- Anxiety disorders
- Substance abuse disorders
- Personality disorders

5.4 Dysthymic Disorder

Dysthymia is a less severe but chronic form of depression that can persist for years with usually moderate intensity.

5.4.1 Diagnosis

Dysthymia (F34.1, 300.4)
Prototypical Symptoms per ICD-10
• Chronic depression of mood which does not currently fulfill the criteria for recurrent depressive disorder, mild or moderate severity (F33.0 or F33.1), in terms of either severity or duration of individual episodes
• Periods of days or weeks of relative wellness may be present, but most of the time (often for months at a time) individual feels tired and depressed, everything is an effort and nothing is enjoyed
• Brooding and complaining, poor sleep, feelings of inadequacy
• Usually able to cope with the basic demands of everyday life
ICD-10 Diagnostic Guidelines
• A very long-standing depression of mood which is never, or only very rarely, severe enough to fulfill the criteria for recurrent depressive disorder, mild or moderate severity (F33.0 or F33.1)
• Rule out bereavement reaction, anxiety, depression. residual schizophrenia
Summary of DMS-10-TR Diagnostic Guidelines
• Depressed mood for most of the day, on most days for least 2 years
• Symptoms include appetite changes, sleeping changes, low energy and fatigue, low self-esteem, poor concentration and indecisiveness, hopelessness
• No history of major depressive episode within 2 years prior to dysthymia onset, or of manic, mixed or hypomanic episodes, or cyclothymic disorder
• Depression does not occur exclusively during the course of a chronic psychotic disorder nor as a result of substance use or abuse or a general medical condition
• The symptoms cause clinically significant distress or impairment in social, occupational, or other important areas of functioning
For exact diagnostic criteria, please refer to the DSM-IV-TR.
DSM-IV-TR Diagnostic Qualifiers
• **Early Onset:** If onset is <21 years • **Late Onset:** If onset is ≥21 years	• **With Atypical Features**

5.4.2 Epidemiology

- Lifetime prevalence: 6%
- Point prevalence: 3%
- Most frequent in females (2:1)

- Dysthymic disorder leads to major depressive disorder in 10%–25% of patients initially diagnosed with dysthymic disorder

5.4.3 Risk Factors

A family history of mood disorders, especially bipolar disorder.

5.4.4 Treatment

- Very poorly studied as compared to major depressive disorder
- Long term psychotherapy (psychodynamic or insight oriented psychotherapy)
- Combined approach including psychotherapy and longer-term use of antidepressants
- Role of antidepressants: SSRIs, MAOIs
- Other psychosocial treatment approaches including vocational counseling

5.5 Bipolar Disorder

5.5.1 Introduction

Bipolar disorder occurs in about 1%-2% of the population. Milder variations of bipolar disorder, such as cyclothymia, may account for another 2%-5%.

5.5.2 Epidemiology

- Lifetime prevalence of classic bipolar disorder is approximately 1%
- The incidence of bipolar disorder is similar in men and women
- The average onset is around 19 years with most cases presenting between 15 and 20 years
- New onset of bipolar disorder is rare after the fifth decade of life
- The prevalence is similar across ethnic groups
- Not generally associated with socioeconomic status

5.5.3 Etiology

- Genetic factors: 1st degree relatives are 7 times more likely to develop the condition than general population (10%-15% risk)
- Neurotransmitter dysregulation: NA, DA< 5HT, glutamine have all been implicated
- Disruption of monoamine signaling and the hypothalamic-pituitary-adrenal axis

5.5.4 Risk Factors

- Alcohol dependence has been associated with an increased risk of manic episodes
- Attention deficit hyperactivity disorder (ADHD)
- Exposure to stimulants and some antidepressants
- Postpartum period

5.5.5   Bipolar Disorder Types and Diagnostic Criteria

Bipolar I Disorder	Bipolar II Disorder
• At least 1 manic episode • May have 1 or more major depressive or mixed episodes	• At least 1 hypomanic episode • At least 1 major depressive episode • May have 1 or more mixed episodes
Cyclothymia	Bipolar Disorder NOS
• At least 1 hypomanic episode • At least 1 depressive episode that doesn't meet the criteria for major depressive episode (dysthymia)	• Does not meet precise criteria of other subtypes

Adapted from the DSM-IV-TR

Bipolar Affective Disorder, Bipolar I/II Disorder (F31.x, 296.xx)*

ICD-10 Diagnostic Guidelines

- **At least 2** episodes in which the patient's mood and activity levels are significantly disturbed, this disturbance consisting on some occasions of manic or hypomanic episodes, and on others of depressive episodes
- **At least 1** of these episodes must be a manic, hypomanic or mixed episode

Summary of DSM-IV-TR Diagnostic Guidelines

Bipolar I Disorder:
- **At least 1 manic or mixed episode**
- Episodes of hypomania or depression may also occur

Bipolar II Disorder:
- **At least 1 hypomanic episode**
- No manic or mixed episodes
- One or more major depressive episodes

*The ICD-10 classification does not have separate categories for Bipolar I and II; Bipolar II is classified under Other bipolar affective disorders (F31.8). Both disorders are classified according to severity, type of manic episode (hypomania or mania), presence of psychosis, etc.

Cyclothymia, Cyclothymic Disorder (F34.0, 301.13)*

ICD-10 Diagnostic Guidelines

- Persistent instability of mood, involving numerous periods of mild depression and mild elation, none of which has been sufficiently severe or prolonged to fulfill the criteria for bipolar affective disorder (F31.x) or recurrent depressive disorder (F33.x)

Cyclothymia, Cyclothymic Disorder (F34.0, 301.13)*
Summary of DSM-IV-TR Diagnostic Guidelines

- Presence of numerous hypomanic and depressive episodes that do not meet criteria for major depressive episode for at least 2 years
- No history of major depressive, manic or mixed episodes during this period
- Not better accounted for by other psychiatric conditions, substance use or a general medical condition

For exact diagnostic criteria, please refer to the DSM-IV-TR.

*ICD-10 classifies mood disorders that are not sufficiently severe or long-lasting to meet the criteria for cyclothymic, dysthymic, bipolar affective or depressive disorders, in a residual category for persistent affective disorders called **Other persistent mood (affective) disorders (F34.8)**.

5.5.6 Features of Bipolar Disease Subtypes

Subtypes	Manic Episode	Hypomanic Episode	Major Depressive Episode (MDE)	Mixed Episode	Dysthymia
Bipolar I	✓	-	Common but not required for diagnosis	✓	-
Bipolar II	-	✓ (At least one episode)	✓ (One or more MDE)	-	-
Bipolar NOS	-	Subthreshold symptoms	Subthreshold symptoms	-	-
Cyclothymic disorder	-	✓	-	-	✓

5.5.7 Definitions of Hypomanic, Manic and Mixed Episodes

Hypomania (F30.0/F31.0, 296.40/296.89)*
Prototypical Symptoms per ICD-10

- Persistent mild elevation of mood (for at least several days), increased energy and activity
- Marked feelings of well-being and both physical and mental efficiency
- Increased sociability, talkativeness, overfamiliarity, increased sexual energy, and a decreased need for sleep
- Irritability, conceit, and boorish behavior may take the place of the more usual euphoric sociability
- Concentration and attention may be impaired, thus diminishing the ability to settle down to work or to relaxation and leisure

Hypomania (F30.0/F31.0, 296.40/296.89)*

ICD-10 Diagnostic Guidelines

- Several of the prototypical symptoms, consistent with elevated or changed mood and increased activity, should be present for **at least several days**
- Considerable, but not severe or total, interference with work or social activity

Summary of DSM-IV-TR Diagnostic Guidelines

- Persistently elevated, expansive, or irritable mood
- Hypomanic symptoms include grandiosity and inflated self-esteem, decreased sleep, pressured speech, flight of ideas and racing thoughts, distractibility, goal-directed activities, involvement in potentially harmful pleasurable activities
- Symptoms are not sufficiently severe to affect occupational or social functioning, require hospitalization or cause psychosis
- Not caused by substance use or a general medical condition

For exact diagnostic criteria, please refer to the DSM-IV-TR.

*The DSM-IV-TR does not have a separate classification for hypomania as a single, separate condition. Hypomanic episodes occur in Bipolar I Disorder, most recent episode hypomanic (296.40) or in Bipolar II disorder (296.89).

Mania Without Psychotic Episode (F30.x/F31.x, 296.0x/296.4x)*

Prototypical Symptoms per ICD-10

- Elevated mood out of keeping with the individual's circumstances and may vary from carefree joviality to almost uncontrollable excitement
- Increased energy, resulting in overactivity, pressure of speech, and a decreased need for sleep
- Normal social inhibitions are lost, attention cannot be sustained, and there is often marked distractibility
- Self-esteem is inflated, grandiose or over-optimistic ideas are freely expressed
- Perceptual disorders may occur, such as the appreciation of colours as especially vivid (and usually beautiful), a preoccupation with fine details of surfaces or textures, and subjective hyperacusis
- The individual may embark on extravagant and impractical schemes, spend money recklessly, or become aggressive, amorous, or facetious in inappropriate circumstances
- The mood may be irritable and suspicious rather than elated

ICD-10 Diagnostic Guidelines

- Mood change accompanied by increased energy and several of the prototypical symptoms (especially pressured speech, decreased need for sleep, grandiosity and excessive optimism) lasting **at least 1 week**
- Severe or complete disruption of occupational and social functioning

Mania Without Psychotic Episode (F30.x/F31.x, 296.0x/296.4x)*
Diagnostic criteria DSM-IV-TR

- A distinct period of abnormally and persistently elevated, expansive, or irritable mood
- Manic symptoms include grandiosity and inflated self-esteem, decreased sleep, pressured speech, flight of ideas and racing thoughts, distractibility, goal-directed activities, involvement in potentially harmful pleasurable activities
- The symptoms do not meet criteria for mixed episode
- Symptoms are sufficiently severe to affect occupational or social functioning, require hospitalization to prevent injury to self or others
- Psychosis is not present
- Not caused by substance use or a general medical condition

For exact diagnostic criteria, please refer to the DSM-IV-TR.

*In ICD-10, mania without psychosis is classified by itself (F30.0) or in Bipolar Affective Disorder (F31.2). The DSM-IV-TR does not have a separate classification for mania by itself. Manic episodes occur in Bipolar I Disorder single manic episode (296.0x) or most recent episode manic (296.4x).

Mania with psychotic episode (F30.2/31.2, 296.04/296.44)*
Prototypical Symptoms per ICD-10

- Same as mania without psychotic episode (F30.1) but more extreme in intensity
- Inflated self-esteem and grandiose ideas may develop into delusions of grandeur, and irritability and suspiciousness into delusions of persecution
- In severe cases, grandiose or religious delusions of identity or role may be prominent, and flight of ideas and pressure of speech may result in the individual becoming incomprehensible
- Severe and sustained physical activity and excitement may result in aggression or violence
- Neglect of eating, drinking, and personal hygiene may result in dangerous states of dehydration and self-neglect

ICD-10 Diagnostic Guidelines

- Severe mood change accompanied by increased energy and several of the prototypical symptoms lasting **at least 1 week**
- Presence of frank psychosis
- Severe or complete disruption of occupational and social functioning

Summary of DSM-IV-TR Diagnostic Guidelines

- Same as mania without psychotic episode
- Frank psychosis is present

For exact diagnostic criteria, please refer to the DSM-IV-TR.

*In ICD-10, mania with psychosis is classified by itself (F30.2) or as part of Bipolar Affective Disorder (F31.2). The DSM-IV-TR does not have a separate classification for mania as a single, separate condition. Manic episodes occur in Bipolar I Disorder single manic episode (296.0x) or most recent episode manic (296.4x).

Mixed Episode (F31.6, 296.6x)*

ICD-10 Diagnostic Guidelines

- A mixture or a rapid alternation of manic, hypomanic, and depressive symptoms lasting **at least 2 weeks**
- Depressive symptoms and symptoms of hypomania or mania may alternate from day to day or even from hour to hour

Summary of DSM-IV-TR Diagnostic Guidelines

- The criteria are met for both a manic episode and a major depressive episode
- Symptoms are sufficiently severe to affect occupational or social functioning, require hospitalization to prevent injury to self or other
- Not caused by substance use or a general medical condition

For exact diagnostic criteria, please refer to the DSM-IV-TR.

*In ICD-10, mixed episodes occur in Bipolar Affective Disorder, current episode mixed (F31.6). In the DSM-IV-TR, mixed episodes occurs in Bipolar I Disorder, most recent episode mixed (296.6x).

5.5.8 Bipolar Episode Specifiers

The DSM-IV-TR uses diagnostic specifiers to further characterize features of bipolar disorder episodes or the overall course or pattern of the disease.

Bipolar Disorder Feature Specifiers (DSM-IV-TR)	
Specifier	Comments
Severity	Mild, moderate, or severe
With Psychosis (for severe episodes)	With or without psychotic symptoms
Remission	In partial or full remission
Chronic	Applied to mood disorder with a major depressive episode
Catatonic	• Motor immobility or excessive purposeless motor activity • Extreme negativism • Peculiarities of voluntary movement • Echolalia
With Melancholic Features*	Cannot experience positive moods, even in the presence of positive events
With Atypical Features*	Mood reactivity (able to experience improved mood in response to positive events)
With Postpartum Onset	Postpartum
*Specifier should be used only if the current or most recent episode is a MDE (the others may be used in manic/hypomanic, mixed, or major depressive episodes)	

Bipolar Disorder Course Specifiers	
Specifier	**Comments**
Longitudinal Course	With or without full interepisode recovery
With Seasonal Pattern*	• Symptoms wax and wane with seasons • More common in bipolar II
With Rapid Cycling*	• 4 or more manic/hypomanic, MDE, or mixed episode in 12 months • More common in bipolar II

*Specifier should be used only if the current or most recent episode is a MDE (the others may be used in manic/hypomanic, mixed, or major depressive episodes)

5.5.9 Tools & Scales

Clinical Interviewing Tools For Diagnosing Bipolar Disorder:
• The Schedule for Affective Disorders and Schizophrenia (SADS)
• Diagnostic Interview Schedule (DIS)
• The Structured Clinical Interview for the DSM-IV-TR (SCID)

Clinician Administered Observational Rating Scales:

Young Mania Rating Scale (YMRS, mod. per Young)										Pts.
Elevated Mood	Absent	0	Mild increase	1	Optimistic, self-confident	2	Elevated, inappropriate	3	Euphoric, inappropriate laughter	4	0-4
Increased Motor Activity, Energy	Absent	0	Subjectively increased	1	Animated	2	Restless, can be calmed	3	Continuous hyperactivity	4	0-4
Sexual Interest	Normal	0	Mild increase	1	Definite increase	2	Spontaneous sex. content	3	overt sexual acts	4	0-4
Sleep	No decrease	0	less, by up to 1 h	1	less by > 1 h	2	decreased need for sleep	3	denies need for sleep	4	0-4
Irritability	Absent	0	subjectively increased	2	irritable at times	4	frequently irritable	6	hostile, uncooperative	8	0-8

Young Mania Rating Scale (cont.)										Pts.
Speech (Rate + Amount)	no increase	0	feels talkative	2	increased rate and amount	4	consistently incr.; pushing	6	pressured; un-interrupt.	8	0-8
Language Thought Disord	absent	0	mildly distractible	1	distractible; loses goal	2	flight of ideas	3	-		0-3
Content of Thoughts	normal	0	questionable plans	2	special projects; hyper religious	4	grandiose or paranoid ideas	6	delusions; hallucinations	8	0-8
Disruptive Aggr. Behavior	absent, cooperative	0	sarcastic, loud at times	2	demanding, makes threats	4	threatens, shouts	6	assaultive, destructive	8	0-8
Appearance	appropriate	0	minimally unkempt	1	poorly groomed or overdressed	2	dishevelled; garish; partly clothed	3	completely unkempt or decorated	4	0-4
Insight	present; admits ill	0	admits possibly ill	1	change in behavior but denies illness	2	possible behavior change	3	denies any behavior change	4	0-4

Manic Rating Scale Score = point total for all 11 parameters
Minimum score: 0, **Maximum score**: 59
Score correlates strongly with severity of mania

- Clinician Administered Rating Scales for Mania (CARS-M)
- Hamilton Depression Rating Scale (HAM-D)
- Montgomery-Asberg Depression Rating Scale (MADRS)
- Inventory of Depressive Symptomatology - Clinician Rated (IDS-C)

Self Rating Scales [8]
- Life chart method
- Internal State Scale (ISS)
- Mood Disorders Questionnaire (MDQ)

Screening for Mania – The Mood Disorder Questionnaire	Yes	No
1. Has there ever been a period of time when you were not your usual self and...		
... you felt so good or so hyper that other people thought you were not your normal self or you were so hyper that you got into trouble?		
... you were so irritable that you shouted at people or started fights or arguments?		
... you felt much more self-confident than usual?		
... you got much less sleep than usual and found you didn‚Äôt really miss it?		
... you were much more talkative or spoke much faster than usual?		
... thoughts raced through your head or you couldn‚Äôt slow your mind down?		
... you were so easily distracted by things around you that you had trouble concentrating or staying on track?		
... you had much more energy than usual?		
... you were much more active or did many more things than usual?		
... you were much more social or outgoing than usual, for example, you telephoned friends in the middle of the night?		
... you were much more interested in sex than usual?		
... you did things that were unusual for you or that other people might have thought were excessive, foolish, or risky?		
... you spent so much money that you got yourself or your family into trouble?		
2. If you checked YES to more than 1 of the above, have several of these ever happened during the same period of time?		
3. How much of a problem did any of these cause you ‚Äì like being unable to work; having family, money or legal troubles; getting into arguments or fights? Please circle one response only		
No Problem Minor Problem Moderate Problem Serious Problem		

Positive screen, if patient answers Yes to 7 or more of the 13 items in question No. 1 AND Yes to question No. 2 AND Moderate or Serious to question No. 3

5.5.10 Bipolar I Disorder

Introduction

- Most of the manic episodes occur before or just after a depressive episode
- Substance abuse is very common
- Earlier age of onset of the first bipolar episode correlates with increased chronicity and overall greater functional impairment
- Untreated manic episode typically lasts 3-4 months and a bipolar depressive episode typically lasts 6-9 months

Differential Diagnosis

Psychiatric Disorders:
- Attention deficit hyperactivity disorder (ADHD)
- Anxiety disorders
- Conduct disorders
- Personality disorders
- Schizophrenia and other psychotic disorders
- Substance use disorders

General Medical Conditions:
- Endocrine disorders
- Infective/inflammatory conditions
- Neurologic disorders
- Metabolic deficiencies

Pharmacological Causes

Investigations

- Full physical examination
- Routine blood tests to exclude any treatable cause: CBC, glucose, electrolytes, calcium, TFTs, LFTs, drug screen, EKG, creatinine clearance

Comorbid Conditions

- Substance abuse (60%)
- Anxiety disorders (up to 50%)
- Social anxiety disorders
- Panic disorder
- Post-traumatic stress disorder
- ADHD

5.5.11 Treatment of Acute Manic Episodes

First line:
- If severe: Lithium plus atypical antipsychotic or valproate plus atypical antipsychotic
- If less severe: Monotherapy of lithium or atypical antipsychotic or valproate
- Benzodiazepines
- Alternatives: Carbamazepine
- Electroconvulsive therapy (ECT)

If first line fails:
- Add a second first line agent
- Add carbamazepine
- Add/change antipsychotic

5.5.12 Treatment of Depressive Disorders

Initial Management:
- If severely depressed, suicidal or when urgent treatment is necessary consider ECT
- If patient is currently drug-free consider initiation of a mood stabilizer (lithium or valproate)
- If patient is already on prophylaxis, optimize the dose while ensuring the compliance, and check serum levels. Exclude/treat any associated problems
- If depressive symptoms persist, consider addition of an antidepressant or an additional mood stabilizer

5.5.13 Algorithm for Treatment of Bipolar Depression

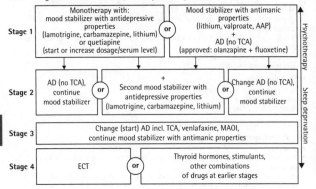

AAP = atypical antipsychotics; AD = antidepressants; ECT = electroconvulsive therapy; MAOI = monoamine oxidase inhibitors; TCA = tricyclic antidepressants

5.5.14 Basic Safety Monitoring for Bipolar Patients

- All patients undergoing treatment for bipolar disorder require medical safety monitoring
- The type and frequency of safety monitoring depends on the specific medication prescribed and also on the individual patient profile and treatment setting. The International Society For Bipolar Disorders (ISBD) recently published consensus guidelines on safety monitoring in bipolar disorder patients. These have the general goals of establishing a baseline prior to treatment initiation, identifying any abnormalities that might influence treatment selection, and screening for medical comorbidities known to be associated with bipolar disorder
- Although the IBSD guidelines do not specify routine monitoring for extrapyramidal symptoms (EPS) including tardive dyskinesia, they do acknowledge that EPS are not uncommonly associated with AAPs. EPS appear to be associated both with dopamine D2 binding affinity as well as rate of dose escalation, target dose, and individual susceptibility factors. Clinicians may choose to systematically assess for EPS using validated scales such as the AIMS, BARS or the Simpson-Angus scale
- Patients on AAPs may also experience metabolic abnormalities (eg, weight gain, hyperglycemia, hyperlipidemia) and pancreatic enzyme elevation
- The table below includes suggested items to be monitored at follow-up:

Monitoring of Patients with Bipolar Depression on Antipsychotics		
History	**Physical Examination**	**Investigations**
Medical • Smoking status • Alcohol intake • Pregnancy potential **Personal/Family** • Cardiovascular disease • Cerebrovascular disease • Hypertension • Dyslipidemia • Diabetes mellitus	• Waist circumference and/or body mass index • Movement abnormalities • Blood pressure	• Complete blood count (Hb/Hct, platelets, WBCs) • Electrolytes • BUN, creatinine • Liver function tests • Amylase, lipase • Spot glucose (fasting if necessary) • Total, LDL, HDL cholesterol • Triglycerides

5.6 Other Mood Disorders

ICD-10 classifies other mood disorders that do not meet the criteria of major depressive or bipolar disorders in a category called Other mood (affective) disorders. This category does not have an exact equivalent in the DSM-IV-TR

Other Mood (Affective) Disorders (F38, -)
Mixed affective episode (F38.00)
• An affective episode lasting for **at least 2 weeks,** characterized by either a mixture or a rapid alternation (usually within a few hours) of hypomanic, manic, and depressive symptoms
Recurrent brief depressive disorder (F38.10)
• Recurrent brief depressive episodes, occurring about once a month over the past year. The individual depressive episodes all last less than 2 weeks (typically 2-3 days, with complete recovery) but fulfill the symptomatic criteria for mild, moderate, or severe depressive episode (F32.0, F32.1, F32.2)
Other specified mood (affective) disorders (F38.8)
• This is a residual category for affective disorders that do not meet the criteria for any other categories F30-F38.1
Unspecified mood (affective) disorder (F38.9)
• To be used only as a last resort, when no other term can be used.

List of references

7   Young RC, Br J Psychiatry 1978; 133:429-433
8   Hirschfeld RM, The Mood Disorder Questionnaire. Prim Care Companion J Clin Psychiatry. 2002 Feb;4(1):9-11
9   Brown G.W and Harris T.O (1978). Social origin of depression: A study of Psychiatric disorders in Women London: Tavistocu publication

6 Delirium

6.1 Introduction

Although classified as a psychiatric disorder delirium is almost always caused by physical disease, head trauma or the effects of drugs. Delirium presents with a fluctuating level of consciousness, and impairment of cognitive, behavioral and emotional functioning.

6.2 Highest Risk Factors

- Increasing age (older than 60 years)
- Associated cognitive impairment (dementia)
- Infection (HIV)
- Burns
- Drug withdrawal
- Use of multiple medications
- Hospitalized ICU patients (up to 80% prevalence)

6.3 Precipitating Factors

I WATCH DEATH acronym
- Infection: Encephalitis, HIV, toxins of drugs, heavy metals
- Withdrawal state: ETOH, sedatives, hypnotics, barbiturates
- Acute metabolic condition: Acid-base and electrolyte imbalance, liver, or renal failure
- Trauma: Brain injury, burns, anemia
- CNS pathology: Hemorrhage, seizure, stroke, tumor
- Hypoxia: CO poisoning, hypoxia, cardiac/pulmonary failure
- Deficiency state: Thiamine, vitamin B12, niacin
- Endocrine problems: Hyperadrenocorticism, hypoadrenocorticism, hyperglycemia, hypoglycemia
- Acute vascular state: Shock
- Toxins of drugs: Pesticides, solvents, many medications
- Heavy metals: Magnesium, lead, mercury

6.4   Clinical Features

Prodromal stage includes symptoms of restlessness, irritability, anxiety and sleep disturbances that develop over a short period of time.

- Symptoms fluctuate during the course of the illness
  - Altered level of consciousness
  - Orientation
  - Agitation
  - Short term memory
  - Hallucinations
- Disturbances in arousal and or psychomotor activity
  - Hyperactive state
  - Hypoactive state
  - Mixed (apathetic, somnolent, withdrawn and quiet, confused)
- Cognitive impairment
  - Memory deficits (cannot register new information)
  - Language disturbance
  - Disorganized thinking →23
  - Disorientation (time of the day, place, date)
- Sleep-wake cycle disturbances
  - Fragmented throughout 24 hour period
  - Reversal sleep (diurnal sleep cycle)
- Altered perceptions
  - Misinterpretation
  - Illusions
  - Hallucinations (visual, auditory, tactile, olfactory) →22
- Delusions
- Affective disturbances
  - Anxiety/fear
  - Depression
  - Irritability
  - Apathy
  - Euphoria
  - Lability of mood
- Neurological abnormalities
  - Tremor
  - Asterixis
  - Myoclonus

6.5 Classification

ICD-10 Classification of Delirium	
Delirium not induced by alcohol or other psychoactive substances (F05)	
F05.0	Delirium, not superimposed on dementia, so described
F05.1	Delirium, superimposed on dementia
F05.8	Other delirium
F05.9	Delirium, unspecified
Delirium due to psychoactive substances*	
F1x.03	Acute intoxication with delirium
F1x.4	Withdrawal state with delirium
F1x.40	With convulsions
F1x.41	Without convulsions
*The first 2 ICD-10 identifiers depend on the particular substance used as follows (F10-F19 in order): alcohol, opioids, cannabinoids, sedative hypnotics, cocaine, stimulants including caffeine, hallucinogens, tobacco, volatile substance, multiple drug use and other psychoactive substances.	
DSM-IV-TR Classification of Delirium	
Dementia related delirium	
290.41	Vascular dementia, with delirium
Intoxication related delirium	
291.0	Alcohol intoxication/withdrawal delirium
292.81	Substance Intoxication/other substance- induced delirium*
Other delirium	
293.0	Delirium due to...[indicate the general medical condition]
780.09	Delirium NOS
*Specify delirium inducing substance, eg, amphetamine, cannabis, cocaine, inhalant, opioid, phencyclidine, sedative hypnotic or anxiolytic intoxication/withdrawal, or unknown/other.	

6.6 Differential Diagnosis of Delirium

- Medical conditions (I WATCHED DEATH) →115
- Psychiatric conditions
  - Dementia
  - Substance induced disorders
  - Mood disorders
  - Psychotic disorders

Unlike these disorders, delirium tends to wax and wane throughout the day. Specific care should be exercised to differentiate delirium from dementia, especially in patients over 60 years of age hospitalized with multiple or serious medical conditions (eg, ICU patients).

Property	Delirium	Dementia
Onset	Rapid (hours to days)	Slow (months to years)
Reversibility	Yes	Typically no
Consciousness	Altered, impaired	Intact
Memory	Impaired	Impaired
Attention	Extremely impaired	Relatively intact (may be impaired in later stages)
Course	Waxes and wanes over the course of the day	Chronic, typically constant over short periods; may express diurnal variation (sundowning)
Causes	Medical (eg, dehydration, drugs, diseases)	Organic brain disease (eg, Alzheimer's, cerebrovascular)
Urgency	Urgent, requires immediate treatment	Chronic, requires chronic management

6.7 Investigations

- Mental status examination
- Performance tests (A tests, Clock Drawing Test, Mini-mental Status Exam (MMSE), Trail A and B)
- Rating Scales
  - Delirium Rating Scales - Revised (DSR-R-98)
  - Confusion Assessment Method (CAM) - 4 item instrument
  - Memorial Delirium Assessment Scale (MDAS) - 10 item scale
  - Delirium Observation Screening scale - 25 item scale

6.8 Diagnostic Workup

- History (including collateral history)
- Physical and cognitive neurological exams
- Vital signs
- Fluid status
- Reviews of medical records
  - Medication review
  - Polypharmacy
  - Drug - drug interaction
  - Toxicity
- Any temporal correlation
- Electrolytes
- BUN
- CBC
- EKG
- CXR
- ABG
- Urinalysis
- Urine drug screening
- Blood alcohol level
- Serum drug levels
- EEG if necessary (low voltage, fast activity)

6.9 Management

- Identify and treat the underlying problem
- Increased observation and monitoring
- Regular monitoring of vital signs and fluid intake and output
- Oxygenation
- Ensure safety from behavioral disturbances
- Coordinate with other physicians
- Facilitate sleep and encourage the return to normal sleep-wake cycles
- Regular lab tests as indicated
- Carefully review all medications and avoid anticholinergic medications; avoid excessive polypharmacy and discontinue medications that are not strictly needed
- Environmental changes
- Provide familiar clues in the environment
- If necessary, use haloperidol or atypical antipsychotics to minimize agitation

7 Dementia

7.1 Definition

The dementias are a heterogeneous group of psychiatric disorders characterized by irreversible global cognitive deficit in the absence of delirium.

7.2 Common Causes of Dementia

- Alzheimer's disease
- Vascular dementia
- Dementia due to other general medical conditions
- Substance induced dementia
- Reversible causes of dementia: Subdural hematoma, NPH, Vitamin B12 deficiency, metabolic causes and hypothyroidism
- Dementia due to multiple etiologies
- Dementia with Lewy bodies

7.3 Classification

ICD-10 Classification of Dementia	
Dementia in Alzheimer's disease (F00)*	
F00.0	With early onset
F00.1	With late onset
F00.2	Atypical or mixed type
F00.9	Unspecified
Vascular dementia (F01)*	
F01.0	Vascular dementia of acute onset
F01.1	Multi-infarct dementia
F01.2	Subcortical vascular dementia
F01.3	Mixed cortical and subcortical vascular dementia
F01.8	Other vascular dementia
F01.9	Vascular dementia, unspecified
Dementia in other diseases classified elsewhere (F02)*	
F02.0	Dementia in Pick's disease
F02.1	Dementia in Creutzfeldt-Jakob disease
F02.2	Dementia in Huntington's disease
F02.3	Dementia in Parkinson's disease

ICD-10 Classification of Dementia	
F02.4	Dementia in human immunodeficiency virus [HIV] disease
F02.8	Dementia in other specified diseases classified elsewhere
Unspecified dementia (F03)	
*5th character specifiers that may be used in Dementia F00–F03	
F0x.x0	Without additional symptoms
F0x.x1	Other symptoms, predominantly delusional
F0x.x2	Other symptoms, predominantly hallucinatory
F0x.x3	Other symptoms, predominantly depressive
F0x.x4	Other mixed symptoms

DSM-IV-TR Classification of Dementia	
Dementia of the Alzheimer's Type	
294.10	With early/late onset, without behavioral disturbance
294.11	With early/late onset, with behavioral disturbance
Vascular dementia[1]	
290.40	Vascular dementia, uncomplicated
290.41	Vascular dementia, with delirium
290.42	Vascular dementia, with delusions
290.43	Vascular dementia, with depressed mood
Substance-induced persisting dementia	
291.2	Alcohol-induced persisting dementia
292.82	Substance-induced persisting dementia[2]
Dementia due to general medical condition[3]	
294.1x	Dementia due to HIV disease
	Dementia due to head trauma
	Dementia due to Parkinson's disease
	Dementia due to Huntington's disease
	Dementia due to Pick's disease
	Dementia due to Creutzfeldt-Jakob disease

[1]Specify if With Behavioral Disturbance
[2]Specify substance: Inhalant; sedative, hypnotic, anxiolytic; or other/unknown
[3]Code presence or absence of a behavioral disturbance in the fifth digit for Dementia Due to a General Medical Condition: 0 =Without Behavioral Disturbance, 1 =With Behavioral Disturbance

7.4 Diagnosis

7.4.1 Core Features

- Multiple cognitive deficits including memory impairment, aphasia, apraxia, agnosia, and disturbances in executive function
- These disturbances cause significant impairment in role functioning and a significant decline from previous level of functioning

7.4.2 ICD-10 Diagnostic Guidelines

ICD-10 Diagnostic Guidelines for Dementia (F00–F03)
Prototypical Symptoms
• Disturbance of multiple higher cortical functions, including memory, thinking, orientation, comprehension, calculation, learning capacity, language, and judgment • Memory dysfunction initially affects registration, storage, and retrieval of new information, but previously learned and familiar material may also be also be lost, particularly in later stages • Impairments of cognitive function are commonly accompanied, and occasionally preceded, by deterioration in emotional control, social behavior, or motivation. • Impairment in the performance of personal activities of daily living, such as washing, dressing, eating, personal hygiene, excretory and toilet activities • Usually chronic and progressive nature • Consciousness is not clouded
General Diagnostic Guidelines
Evidence for **at least 6 months** of the following symptoms: • Decline in both memory and thinking sufficient to impair personal activities of daily living • Impairment of thinking and reasoning capacity, and a reduction in the flow of ideas • Difficulty with processing new information, attending to multiple stimuli at the same time, and shifting focus of attention from one topic to another

ICD-10 Diagnostic Guidelines for Dementia (F00-F03)
Dementia in Alzheimer's Disease (F00)

- Absence of clinical evidence or findings that suggest other causes for the dementia (eg, hypothyroidism, cerebrovascular disease, hypercalcemia, vitamin B12 deficiency, niacin deficiency, neurosyphilis, normal pressure hydrocephalus, or subdural hematoma)
- Absence of a sudden, apoplectic onset, or of neurological signs of focal damage such as hemiparesis, sensory loss, visual field defects, and incoordination occurring early in the illness (although these phenomena may be superimposed later)
- Prominence of features of temporal and parietal lobe damage, including dysphasia or dyspraxia

Subtypes:

- **Early onset (F00.0):**
  - Symptoms of dementia develop **before age 65 years**
  - A **relatively more rapid course** than AD dementia with late onset (>65 years)
- **Late onset (F00.1):**
  - Symptoms of dementia develop **after age 65 years**
  - Relatively more insidious onset and a slower progression and deterioration than early onset AD dementia; usually develops over 2-3 years, but may take longer
  - Other symptoms are as in early onset AD dementia
- **Atypical or mixed type (F00.2):**
  - Symptoms do not fit the descriptions and guidelines for either F00.0 or F00.1

Vascular dementia (F01)

- History of cerebrovascular accidents, stroke, transient ischemic attacks or other symptoms associated with cerebrovascular disease such as hypertension or carotid bruits
- Uneven impairment of cognitive function (memory and intellectual function) and focal neurological signs
- Abrupt onset or stepwise deterioration
- Symptoms may include transient depressive mood, weeping or explosive laughter, and transient episodes of clouded consciousness or delirium, often provoked by further infarction
- Personality changes may occur in a proportion of cases including apathy, disinhibition, or accentuation of previous traits such as egocentricity, paranoid attitudes, or irritability

ICD-10 Diagnostic Guidelines for Dementia (F00–F03)

Subtypes:
- **Vascular dementia of acute onset (F01.0):**
  - Usually develops rapidly after a succession of strokes from cerebrovascular thrombosis, embolism, or hemorrhage
- **Multi-infarct dementia (F01.1):**
  - More gradual in onset than the acute form, following a number of minor ischemic episodes which produce an accumulation of infarcts in the cerebral parenchyma
- **Subcortical vascular dementia (F01.2):**
  - History of hypertension and foci of ischemic destruction in the deep white matter of the cerebral hemispheres
  - Despite relative preservation of the cerebral cortex, symptoms resemble those of Alzheimer's dementia
- **Mixed cortical and subcortical vascular dementia (F01.3):**
Mixed cortical and subcortical clinical features of vascular dementia

Dementia of Pick's Disease (F02.0)

- A progressive dementia, commencing in middle life (**usually between 50 and 60 years**)
- **A predominance of frontal lobe features** with euphoria, emotional blunting, and coarsening of social behavior, disinhibition, and either apathy or restlessness (fewer temporal and parietal features than AD dementia)
- The social and behavioral manifestations often precede frank memory impairment
- Slowly progressing changes of character and social deterioration, followed by impairment of intellect, memory, and language functions, with apathy, euphoria, and (occasionally) extrapyramidal phenomena
- Selective neuropathological atrophy of the frontal and temporal lobes without occurrence of neuritic plaques and neurofibrillary tangles in excess of that seen in normal aging

Dementia in Creutzfeldt-Jakob disease (F02.1)

- Devastating, rapidly progressing dementia (1–2 years) accompanied by multiple neurological symptoms (which may precede the onset of dementia in the amyotrophic form)
- Progressive spastic paralysis of the limbs, accompanied by extrapyramidal signs with tremor, rigidity, and choreoathetoid movements.
- Ataxia, visual failure, or muscle fibrillation and atrophy of the upper motor neuron type
- **Classic triad of symptoms** is highly suggestive of disease:
  - Rapidly progressing, devastating dementia
  - Pyramidal and extrapyramidal disease with myoclonus
  - A characteristic (triphasic) electroencephalogram

ICD-10 Diagnostic Guidelines for Dementia (F00–F03)

Dementia in Huntington's disease (F02.2)

- Symptoms typically emerge in the third and fourth decade of life with slow progression leading to death in 10–15 years
- Involuntary choreiform movements, typically of the face, hands, and shoulders, or in the gait, are early manifestations that usually precede the dementia
- Dementia characterized by the predominant involvement of frontal lobe functions in the early stage, with relative late preservation of memory

Dementia in Parkinson's disease (F02.3)

- A dementia developing in the course of established and advanced Parkinson's disease (especially its severe forms)
- No particular distinguishing clinical features have yet been identified

Dementia in HIV disease (F02.4)

- Typically presents with complaints of forgetfulness, slowness, poor concentration, and difficulties with problem-solving and reading
- Apathy, reduced spontaneity, and social withdrawal are common, and in a significant minority of affected individuals the illness may present atypically with an affective disorder, psychosis, or seizures
- Physical examination often reveals tremor, impaired rapid repetitive movements, imbalance, ataxia, hypertonia, generalized hyperreflexia, positive frontal release signs, and impaired pursuit and saccadic eye movements

Dementia in other specified diseases classified elsewhere (F02.8)

- Dementia as a consequence of a variety of cerebral and somatic conditions.
- Parkinsonism-dementia complex of Guam, also known as Lytico-Bodig disease (rapidly progressing dementia followed by extrapyramidal dysfunction and, in some cases, amyotrophic lateral sclerosis) should be coded here
- Specify the ICD-10 code for the underlying condition

7.4.3　DSM–IV–TR Diagnostic Guidelines

Summary of DSM–IV–TR Diagnostic Guidelines for Dementia

Dementia of the Alzheimer's type (294.10/294.11)

- **Memory impairment** and cognitive defects such as apraxia, aphasia, agnosia or impaired executive functioning
- Symptoms cause significant occupational/social functioning decline, are gradual in onset, and progressive in course
- Not caused by other conditions known to cause dementia (eg, cerebrovascular disease, Parkinson Disease, Huntington Disease, tumors, etc), a systemic medical condition, or intoxication
- Does not occur exclusively during delirium and is not better explained by another axis I disorder (eg, major depressive disorder)
- **Subtypes:**
  - **Without behavioral disturbance (294.10)**
  - **With behavioral disturbance (294.11):** eg, wandering, agitation

For exact diagnostic criteria, please refer to the DSM–IV–TR.

7.5　Anatomical Classification

Cortical Dementia	Subcortical Dementia
• Dementia of the Alzheimer's type	• Dementia due to HIV
• Fronto-temporal dementia	• Dementia due to Parkinson's disease
• Dementia due to Creutzfeldt-Jakob disease (CJD)	• Dementia due to Huntington's disease
• Dementia due to chronic subdural hematoma	• Dementia due to multiple sclerosis

7.6　Differential Diagnosis of Dementia

- Delirium
- Mood disorder (eg, depression)
- Substance use disorders
- Psychotic disorder
- Normal aging
- Mental retardation

7.7 Medical Workup

- CBC
- Electrolytes including calcium, magnesium, phosphate
- BUN, creatinine, glucose
- Liver function tests
- Vitamin B12, folate
- Erythrocyte sedimentation rate
- Thyroid profile with TSH
- ECG
- Chest X-ray
- Syphilis serology (if necessary)
- Urine analysis and urine toxicology
- Other imaging studies such as CT, MRI or SPECT
- Lumbar puncture and CSF analysis/culture
- Blood culture
- Depending on type of dementia, other investigations may be warranted

7.8 Principles of Management

- Detailed assessment to control diagnosis
- Identify the type of dementia
- Consider cognitive enhancers (eg, acetylcholinesterase inhibitors, NMDA receptor partial antagonist)
- Identify and treat other comorbid psychiatric conditions, especially depression
- Symptomatic treatment for depression insomnia and other behavioral disturbances
- Psychological support and illness education for caregivers
- Social management
- If identifiable cause is present, recommend treatment

8 Personality Disorders

8.1 General Information

Personality disorders are common in community and clinical settings. These disorders can cause significant problems for sufferers and their close ones, are costly to society, and can complicate the treatment of other psychiatric disorders. The goal of identifying personality disorders is to understand their influence on the physical and emotional well-being of individuals.

Personality traits vs personality disorders
Personality traits are normal, flexible, adaptive patterns of relating to the environment. Personality traits vary considerably, but are considered normal for a given cultural and social environment, and do not cause personal emotional distress or a decrease in functioning. On the other hand, personality disorders are traits that have become amplified or exaggerated, inflexible, enduring, maladaptive, and distress provoking. They typically emerge in early childhood or adolescence.

Dramatic changes in personality are unexpected and may be a sign of other more acute pathology, such as organic disease, dementia or another neuropsychiatric disorder.

8.2 Prevalence

Personality disorders are highly prevalent. About 10%-15% of the general population has at least one personality disorder. Among psychiatric patients, outpatient prevalence is about 30%-50%, while inpatient prevalence is >50%. Among patients with Axis I disorders, one third have comorbid personality disorders.

8.3 Etiology

Exact etiology is unknown. There is likely interplay of genetic, biological, environmental, and developmental factors.

8.4 Classification of Personality Disorders

ICD-10 Classification of Personality Disorders	
Specific personality disorders (F60)	
F60.0	Paranoid personality disorder
F60.1	Schizoid personality disorder
F60.2	Dissocial personality disorder
F60.3	Emotionally unstable personality disorder
F60.30	Impulsive type
F60.31	Borderline type
F60.4	Histrionic personality disorder
F60.5	Anankastic personality disorder
F60.6	Anxious (avoidant) personality disorder
F60.7	Dependent personality disorder
F60.8	Other specific personality disorder
F60.9	Personality disorder, unspecified
Mixed and other personality disorders (F61)	
F61.0	Mixed personality disorders
F61.1	Troublesome personality changes
Enduring personality changes, not attributable to brain damage/disease (F62.x)	
F62.0	Enduring personality change after catastrophic experience
F62.1	Enduring personality change after psychiatric illness
F62.8	Other enduring personality changes
F62.9	Enduring personality change, unspecified
DSM-IV-TR Classification of Personality Disorders (Axis II)	
Cluster A personality disorders: Odd or eccentric	
301.0	Paranoid personality disorder
301.20	Schizoid personality disorder
301.22	Schizotypal personality disorder
Cluster B personality disorders: Dramatic, emotional or erratic	
301.7	Antisocial personality disorder
301.83	Borderline personality disorder
301.50	Histrionic personality disorder
301.81	Narcissistic personality disorder
Cluster A personality disorders: Anxious or fearful	
301.82	Avoidant personality disorder

DSM-IV-TR Classification of Personality Disorders (Axis II)	
301.6	Dependent personality disorder
301.4	Obsessive-compulsive personality disorder
Other personality disorders	
301.9	Personality disorder not otherwise specified
310.1	Personality change due to a general medical condition

8.5 Diagnosis

8.5.1 General Diagnostic Guidelines

ICD-10 Diagnostic Guidelines for Specific Personality Disorders (F60)

Conditions not directly attributable to gross brain damage or disease, or to another psychiatric disorder, meeting the following criteria:

- Markedly disharmonious attitudes and behavior, involving usually several areas of functioning, eg, affectivity, arousal, impulse control, ways of perceiving and thinking, and style of relating to others
- The abnormal behavior pattern is enduring, of long standing, and not limited to episodes of mental illness
- The abnormal behavior pattern is pervasive and clearly maladaptive to a broad range of personal and social situations
- The above manifestations always appear during childhood or adolescence and continue into adulthood
- The disorder leads to considerable personal distress but this may only become apparent late in its course
- The disorder is usually, but not invariably, associated with significant problems in occupational and social performance

For different cultures it may be necessary to develop specific sets of criteria with regard to social norms, rules and obligations.

Summary of DSM-IV-TR Diagnostic Guidelines for Personality Disorder

- A personality disorder is an internal experience and behavior that is markedly different from cultural norms as manifested through cognition, affectivity, interpersonal functioning and impulse control
- This pattern starts in adolescence or early adulthood, is enduring, inflexible, and causes significant distress and impairment across a wide range of activities and functioning
- The disorder is not better explained by an Axis I condition, substance use or a medical condition

For exact diagnostic criteria, please refer to the DSM-IV-TR.

8.5.2 Testing for personality disorders

- Personality disorders are difficult to diagnose
  - Obtain longitudinal history, multiple areas of functioning, and collateral data
  - Self-report instruments: Personality diagnostic inventory (PDQ), Wisconsin Personality Disorders Inventory (WISPI-IV)
- Objective Tests:
  - Minnesota Multiphasic Personality Inventory-II (MMPI-II): Consists of 567 true-false questions
  - Million Clinical Multiaxial Inventory-III (MCMI-III): Consists of 157 true-false questions
  - Borderline Personality Organization Scale
  - Narcissistic Personality Inventory
- Projective Tests:
  - Thematic Apperception Test
  - Rorschach (inkblot) Test

8.6 Defense Mechanisms

Defense mechanisms are unconscious processes used to reduce anxiety when uncomfortable and unpleasant emotions arise. Defense mechanisms can be classified into following broad categories.

8.6.1 Classification

Mature	Immature	Neurotic	Psychotic
• Altruism • Asceticism • Suppression • Anticipation • Affiliation • Humor	• Acting out • Idealization/ devaluation • Projection • Dissociation	• Repression • Rationalization • Isolation • Reaction formation • Denial • Dissociation • Displacement	• Distortion of external reality • Denial of external reality

8.6.2 Mature

- **Altruism:** Selfless concern for welfare of others. Suppressing an emotion by doing something good for others
- **Asceticism:** Eliminating the pleasurable effects of experience
- **Suppression:** Consciously or semiconsciously postponing attention to a conscious impulse or conflict. Sublimation-Impulses directed to socially useful projects
- **Anticipation:** Realistically anticipating or planning for future inner discomfort
- **Affiliation:** Seeking out others for emotional or physical support
- **Humor:** Noticing the amusing or ironic aspects of something rather than the unpleasant aspects

8.6.3 Immature

- **Acting out:** Expressing an emotion in an action rather than keeping it in awareness
- **Idealization/devaluation (splitting):** Person or object is viewed as either all good or all bad (borderline PD)
- **Projection:** Attributing unacknowledged anger and feelings to others
- **Dissociation:** Dissociating instead of feeling the pain

8.6.4 Neurotic

- **Repression:** Removing the emotion out of conscious awareness
- **Rationalization:** Coming with a convincing, but usually false reason why you are not bothered
- **Isolation**
- **Reaction formation:** Transforming an unacceptable impulse into its opposite
- **Denial:** Denial of the existence of painful thoughts
- **Dissociation:** Unpleasant affects are replaced with pleasant ones
- **Displacement:** Shifting an affect from one person or object to another

8.6.5 Psychotic

- Distortion of external reality, denial of external reality

8.6.6 Treatment

- Persons often resist treatment
- Psychotherapy is the treatment of choice
- Medications can be used for comorbid Axis I symptoms or disorders
- Caregiver psychoeducation about how to manage affects/behaviors

8.7 Paranoid Personality Disorder

8.7.1 Prevalence

Prevalence rate is ~ 4% in general population. They are more common in males. There is increased prevalence in new immigrants, minority groups, and the hearing impaired.

8.7.2 Core Features

- Pervasive mistrust and extreme suspiciousness, but not of delusional proportions; distrust of others, others' motives interpreted as malevolent
- Mnemonic: **SUSPECT** (need 4 of the following 7 criteria):
  - **S**pouse infidelity suspected
  - **U**nforgiving
  - **S**uspicious of others
  - **P**erceives slights/attacks
  - **E**nemy or friend (have doubts of the loyalty of friends or associates)
  - **C**onfiding in others difficult because of fear of betrayal
  - **T**hreats perceived in benign event

8.7.3 Psychological Defenses

- Projection, projective identification, denial, and rationalization

8.7.4 Treatment

- Supportive therapy to help individuals navigate life. Cognitive behavioral therapy to challenge their paranoid beliefs
- Medications can be used to treat comorbidities

8.8 Schizoid Personality Disorder

8.8.1 Prevalence

It affects ~ 3% of the general population. Male female ratio is approx. 2:1

8.8.2 Core Features

- Detached from relationships, restricted range of emotional expression
- Mnemonic: **DISTANT** (need 4 of the following 7 criteria)
  - **D**etached affect
  - **I**ndifferent to praise and criticism
  - **S**exual experiences of little interest
  - **T**asks done solitary
  - **A**bsence of close friends
  - **N**either desires nor enjoys close relatives
  - **T**akes pleasure in few activities

8.8.3 Psychological Defenses

- Fantasy, projection, intellectualization

8.8.4 Treatment

- Individual supportive and cognitive therapy
- Social skill and assertiveness training
- Medications can be used to treat the comorbidities

8.9   Schizotypal Personality Disorder

8.9.1   Prevalence

It affects ~ 2%-5% of the general population. It is more common in males

8.9.2   Core Features

- Acute discomfort with and decreased capacity for close relationships, cognitive and perception distortions, and eccentric behavior
- Mnemonic: **ME PECULIAR** (need 5 of the following 10 criteria)
  - **M**agical thinking or odd beliefs
  - **E**xperiences unusual perceptions
  - **P**aranoid ideation
  - **E**ccentric behavior or appearance
  - **C**onstricted or inappropriate affect
  - **U**nusual (odd) thinking and speech
  - **L**acks close friends
  - **I**deas of reference
  - **A**nxiety in social situations
  - **R**ule out psychotic disorder and pervasive developmental disorder

8.9.3   Psychological Defenses

Projection, denial, distortion

8.9.4   Treatment

- Individual support (monitor for suicide and decompensation into psychosis) and cognitive therapy (to address misperceptions and overvalued ideas)
- Social skill and assertiveness training
- Medications can be used to treat the comorbidities
- About 10% of the patients with this disorder eventually commit suicide

8.10 Antisocial Personality Disorder

8.10.1 Prevalence

- It affects 3%-4% of males and 1% of the females
- Previously classified as sociopaths or psychopaths. They rarely seek help for distress caused by their actions. Most common reasons for psychiatric contact include seeking prescription with a street value, detox, notes for missing work, assessment to relieve them of criminal responsibility.

8.10.2 Core Features

- Disregard and violation of rights of others since age 15 of years. Do not diagnose until the age of 18 years
- Mnemonic: **CORRUPT** (need 3 out of the following 7 criteria)
    - **C**onformity to law lacking
    - **O**bligations ignored
    - **R**eckless disregard for the safety of self or others
    - **R**emorse lacking
    - **U**nderhanded (deceitful, lies, cons others)
    - **P**lanning insufficient (impulsive)
    - **T**emper (irritable and aggressive)

8.10.3 Psychological Defenses

Acting out, projection, isolation of affect, somatization, dissociation

8.10.4 Treatment

No form of treatment has been shown to be consistently effective
- Group therapy - homogenous with peer confrontation appears to be most effective. Develop clear treatment contract. Provide clear limit setting and boundaries
- Medications can be used to treat the comorbidities. Avoid prescribing medications with street value

8.11 Borderline Personality Disorder

8.11.1 Prevalence

Prevalence is 2.5% of the general population, accounting for half of all people with personality disorders. It is present in 10% of psychiatric outpatients and 20% of inpatients. It is three times more common in women. Prevalence decreases with age. A history of childhood sexual or physical trauma is often present in persons with borderline personality disorder.

8.11.2 Core Features

- Instability of self-image, relationships, affect, with impulsivity
- Mnemonic: **AM SUICIDE** (need 5 of the following 9 criteria)
  - **A**bandonment
  - **M**ood instability
  - **S**uicidal behavior, gestures, or threats, or self-injurious behavior
  - **U**nstable and intense interpersonal relationships
  - **I**mpulsivity in two potentially damaging areas
  - **C**ontrolling anger is difficult
  - **I**dentity disturbance
  - **D**issociative or paranoid symptoms that are transient and stress related
  - **E**mptiness

8.11.3 Psychological Defenses

Projective identification, splitting, dissociation, denial, and distortion

8.11.4 Treatment

- Psychotherapy is the cornerstone of treatment. These individuals are a challenge to treat. They are very willing to be treated and readily attach to the therapist. Individual, group, and family therapy can be useful. Dialectical behavioral therapy - teaches patients to improve coping skills, fundamental skills training, help patients learn to appropriately manage anger and tolerate stress. Cognitive behavioral therapy, and psychodynamic therapy (transference based therapy) can also be used to treat patients with this personality disorder
- Medications can help with affective dysregulation, impulsivity/aggression, and cognitive/perceptual symptoms
- Hospitalization: Short-term hospitalization with clear achievable goals can be considered for life-threatening suicide attempt or immediate danger to others, persistent depression, transient psychosis, relapse into drug abuse. While hospitalized, close communication between staff is essential to avoid splitting. Setting firm limits, and consistent treatment plan is also essential

8.12 Histrionic Personality Disorder

8.12.1 Prevalence

Prevalence rates are about 2% in the general population. More common in women.

8.12.2 Core Features

- Excessive emotionality and attention seeking
- Mnemonic: **PRAISE ME** (need 5 of the following 8 criteria)
  - **P**rovocative (or sexually seductive behavior)
  - **R**elationships considered more intimate than they are
  - **A**ttention (uncomfortable when not the center of attention)
  - **I**nfluenced easily
  - **S**tyle of speech (wants to impress, lacks detail)
  - **E**motions (rapidly shifting and shallow)
  - **M**ade up (physical appearance used to draw attention to self)
  - **E**motions exaggerated - theatrical

8.12.3 Treatment

- Individual, group, and behavioral therapy are the treatment of choice
- Medications can be used to treat the comorbidities

8.13 Narcissistic Personality Disorder

8.13.1 Prevalence

Prevalence rates are less than 1%. It is more common in males.

8.13.2 Core Features

- Grandiosity, need for admiration, and lack of empathy
- Mnemonic: **SPEEECIAL** (need 5 of the following 9 criteria)
  - **S**pecial (believes he or she is special)
  - **P**reoccupied with fantasies of unlimited power, success
  - **E**nvious of others or believes that are envious of him
  - **E**ntitlement
  - **E**xcess admiration required
  - **C**onceited
  - **I**nterpersonal exploitation
  - **A**rrogant, haughty

8.13.3 Psychological Defenses

- Identification, projection, splitting

8.13.4 Treatment

- Individual psychodynamic and cognitive therapy. People with this disorder do not tolerate group settings well
- Medications can be used for affective instability

8.14 Avoidant Personality Disorder

8.14.1 Prevalence

Prevalence rates are 2%-3% in the general population. This disorder is more common in females

8.14.2 Core Features

- Social inhibition, feeling of inadequacy, hypersensitivity to negative evaluation
- Mnemonic: **CRINGES** (need 4 of the following 7 criteria)
  - **C**ertainty of being liked required before willing to risk involvement
  - **R**ejection preoccupies person's thoughts in social situations
  - **I**ntimate relationships are avoided
  - **N**ew relationships inhibited or avoided
  - **G**ets around occupational activities that involve interpersonal contact
  - **E**mbarrassment potential prevents new activity or taking personal risks
  - **S**elf-viewed as unappealing, inept, and inferior

8.14.3 Psychological Defenses

- Avoidance, inhibition, isolation of affect, projection, displacement

8.14.4 Treatment

- Individual, group, cognitive behavioral therapy, and family therapy are the treatment of choice. Individuals are likely to have the best response of all the personality disorders to psychotherapy
- Medications can be used to treat the comorbidities

8.15 Dependent Personality Disorder

8.15.1 Prevalence

Prevalence rates in the general population are 2%-4%. This disorder is more common in females

8.15.2 Core features

- Pervasive, excessive need to be taken care of, submissive, clinging behavior, and fear of separation
- Mnemonic: **RELIANCE** (need 5 of the following 8 criteria)
  - **R**eassurance needed for decisions
  - **E**xpressing disagreement is difficult due to the fear of loss of support or approval
  - **L**ife responsibilities assumed by others
  - **I**nitiating projects is difficult due to lack of self-confidence
  - **A**lone, feels helpless and a sense of discomfort when alone
  - **N**urturance, goes to great lengths to obtain nurturance and support
  - **C**ompanionship sought urgently when close relationship ends
  - **E**xaggerated fears of being left to care for self

8.15.3 Psychological Defenses

- Idealization, somatization, reaction formation, and projective identification
- Predisposing factors: Include childhood separation, anxiety, abuse, or chronic illness

8.15.4 Treatment

- Individual and group psychotherapy
- Cognitive behavioral therapy with assertiveness skill training
- Medications can be used to treat the comorbidities

8.16 Obsessive-Compulsive Personality Disorder

8.16.1 Prevalence

This is the most prevalent personality disorder. Prevalence rates are about 8% in the general population. There is no difference in frequency between males and females.

8.16.2 Core Features

- Orderliness, mental and interpersonal control, perfectionism, at the expense of flexibility, openness, and efficiency
- Mnemonic: **LAW FIRMS** (need 4 of the following 8 criteria)
  - **L**oses point of activity due to preoccupation with detail
  - **A**bility to complete tasks is compromised by perfectionism
  - **W**orthless objects unable to discard
  - **F**riendships and leisure activities excluded due to preoccupation with work
  - **I**nflexible, unscrupulous, over conscientious on ethics, values, or morality, not accounted for by religion or culture
  - **R**eluctant to delegate unless others submit to exact guidelines
  - **M**iserly toward self and others
  - **S**tubbornness and rigidity

8.16.3 Psychological Defenses

- Reaction formation, undoing, isolation of affect, intellectualization

8.16.4 Treatment

- Cognitive behavioral therapy is the treatment of choice
- Medications can be used to treat the comorbidities

8.17 Personality Disorder Not Otherwise Specified

- Personality dysfunction which does not meet full criteria for one specific personality disorder
- Specific personality types in NOS category
  - **Passive–Aggressive PD:** Lack assertiveness, passively resist demands on self, finds faults, delays/procrastinates, and complains without action
  - **Depressive PD:** Negative, pessimistic, broody, negative self-evaluation, negative view of others, anhedonic, unhappy

8.18 Personality Change due to a General Medical Condition (GMC)

- **Labile type:** Affective lability
- **Disinhibited type:** Poor impulse control
- **Aggressive type:** Aggressive type
- **Apathetic type:** Apathy and indifference
- **Paranoid type:** Suspiciousness and paranoia
- **Other type, combined type, unspecified type:** Epilepsy syndrome - religiosity, hyposexuality, humorlessness, stickiness, periodic rage and paranoia

9 Impulse Control Disorders

9.1 Introduction

Impulse control disorders are behavioral impulse-related disorders that are not classified elsewhere. These disorders are characterized by recurrent acts with no clear rational motivation that generally harm the patient's own interests and those of others. Patients report that the behavior is associated with impulses to action that cannot be controlled.

9.2 Classification

ICD-10 Classification of Habit and Impulse Disorders (F63)	
F63.0	Pathological gambling
F63.1	Pathological fire-setting (pyromania)
F63.2	Pathological stealing (kleptomania)
F63.3	Trichotillomania
F63.8	Other habit and impulse disorders
F63.9	Habit and impulse disorder, unspecified
DSM-IV-TR Classification of Impulse Control Disorders (312)	
312.30	Impulse-control disorder NOS
312.31	Pathological gambling
312.32	Kleptomania
312.33	Pyromania
312.34	Intermittent explosive disorder
312.39	Trichotillomania

9.3 Intermittent Explosive Disorder

9.3.1 Diagnosis

ICD-10 Diagnostic Guidelines (F63.8)

The ICD-10 does not have a separate category for this condition. Intermittent Explosive Disorder should be classified under **Other habit and impulse disorders (F63.8).** These disorders are generally characterized by the following features:

- Persistent maladaptive behavior that is not secondary to a recognized psychiatric syndrome
- Repeated failure to resist impulses to carry out the behavior.
- A prodromal period of tension with a feeling of release at the time of the act.

Summary of DSM-IV-TR Diagnostic Guidelines (312.34)

Tendency for violent and grossly disproportionate responses to aggressive impulses resulting in repeated acts of assault or property destruction.
For exact diagnostic criteria, please refer to the DSM-IV-TR.

9.3.2 Epidemiology

- Underreported, but is thought to be extremely rare
- Is more prevalent in males compared to females
- Is potentially more common in first degree biological relatives of persons with the disorder

9.3.3 Etiology

- Psychosocial factors: An unfavorable childhood environment filled with alcohol dependence, violence and threats to life
- Adverse events in infancy and childhood, such as perinatal trauma, infantile seizures, head trauma, encephalitis, minimal brain dysfunction and hyperactivity
- Biological factors: Decreased serotonergic activity in the limbic system or high testosterone concentration in the CSF may predispose to lack of behavioral inhibition

9.3.4 Course

- Onset can be sudden or insidious; limited data suggests Intermittent Explosive Disorder may appear from childhood to the early 20s
- Course can be episodic or chronic

9.3.5   Differential Diagnosis

- Psychotic disorders
- Personality change secondary to a general medical condition
- Antisocial personality disorder
- Borderline personality disorder
- Substance intoxication or withdrawal
- Epilepsy
- Brain tumors
- Degenerative diseases
- Delirium, dementia
- Endocrine disorders
- Conduct disorder
- Oppositional defiant disorder
- Manic episode
- Major depressive disorder
- Panic disorder
- Malingering
- *Amok*, traditionally reported in southeastern Asia, is characterized by a single episode of acute violent behavior associated with amnesia for the event and prominent dissociative features

9.3.6   Treatment

- Psychotherapy, including group and family therapy
- Anticonvulsants
- Antipsychotics
- Tricyclic drugs
- SSRIs
- Beta-adrenergic receptor antagonists (eg, propranolol)
- Calcium channel inhibitors

9.3.7   Comorbidities

- Other impulse control disorders
- Substance use
- Mood disorder
- Anxiety disorders
- Eating disorders
- High rates of fire setting have been reported

9.4 Kleptomania

9.4.1 Diagnosis

ICD-10 Diagnostic Guidelines (F63.2)

- Repeated failure to resist impulses to steal objects that are not acquired for personal use or monetary gain; objects may instead be discarded, given away, or hoarded
- Increasing sense of tension before, and a sense of gratification during and immediately after, the act
- The theft is a solitary act, not carried out with an accomplice, and full efforts for concealment are not always undertaken
- Individual may express anxiety, despondency, and guilt between episodes of stealing, but this does not prevent repetition

Summary of DSM-IV-TR Diagnostic Guidelines (312.32)

- Recurrent failure to resist impulse to steal objects that are not needed for personal use or monetary value
- There's a sense of tension prior to the act of stealing and a sense of relief and gratification when committing the act
- Act should not be driven by anger or revenge, or caused by other psychiatric disorders

For exact diagnostic criteria, please refer to the DSM-IV-TR.

9.4.2 Epidemiology

- Kleptomania is rare, with an estimated prevalence of 0.6%, occurring in less than 5% of identified shoplifters
- Approximately 2/3 of those with the disorder are female

9.4.3 Etiology

- Emergence of Kleptomania often occurs during times of significant stress, including losses, separations and endings of important relationships
- Brain diseases and mental retardation, focal neurological signs, cortical atrophy and enlarged lateral ventricles have been noted in some patients
- Genetic factors are suggested by an increased incidence of Kleptomania in patients with first degree relatives with obsessive compulsive disorder and mood disorders

9.4.4 Course

Variable age of onset

Course	Stealing Episodes	Periods of Remission
Sporadic	Brief	Long
Episodic	Protracted	Protracted
Chronic (most common)	Fluctuate	Fluctuate

9.4.5 Differential Diagnosis

- Ordinary acts of theft or shoplifting (act is deliberate, motivated by the stolen object or a response to social pressures eg, response to a dare, act of rebellion, rite of passage)
- Antisocial personality disorder
- Conduct disorder
- Intentional or inadvertent stealing during manic episodes
- Response to delusions or hallucinations (eg, schizophrenia)
- Dementia

9.4.6 Treatment

- Insight oriented therapy, psychoanalysis
- Behavior therapy (including systematic desensitization, aversive conditioning, +/- altered social contingencies)
- SSRIs (fluoxetine, fluvoxamine)
- Tricyclics
- Trazodone
- Lithium
- Valproic acid
- Naltrexone

9.5 Pyromania

9.5.1 Diagnosis

ICD-10 Diagnostic Guidelines (F63.1)

- Repeated fire-setting without any obvious motive such as monetary gain, revenge, or political extremism
- An intense interest in watching fires burn
- Reported feelings of increasing tension before the act, and intense excitement immediately after it has been carried out
- Deliberate fire-setting due to motive, conduct disorder, personality disorder or other psychiatric or organic condition should be ruled out

---

Summary of DSM-IV-TR Diagnostic Guidelines (312.33)

- Repeated fire setting characterized by tension and emotional arousal prior to act and gratification and relief during and after the act
- Fascination with fires, situations and objects associated with fires
- Must rule out motive such as criminal activity concealment, revenge, financial motives, impaired judgment or other personality or psychiatric disorders

For exact diagnostic criteria, please refer to the DSM-IV-TR.

9.5.2 Epidemiology

Pyromania is rare; occurs far more often in men than women.

9.5.3 Risk Factors

Further studies are needed to elucidate risk factors.

9.5.4 Course

- Unknown typical age of onset or longitudinal course
- Fire-setting incidents tend to be episodic and may wax and wane in frequency

9.5.5 Differential Diagnosis

- Intentional fire setting for profit, sabotage, or revenge; to conceal a crime; to make a political statement; or to attract attention or recognition
- Developmental experimentation in childhood
- Conduct disorder
- Antisocial personality disorder
- Manic episode
- Schizophrenia
- Dementia
- Mental retardation
- Substance intoxication

9.5.6 Treatment

Difficult to treat given the perpetrator's lack of motivation. No single treatment has been proven to be effective. Incarceration to prevent recurrence with subsequent behavior therapy may be effective.

9.5.7 Comorbidities

- Alcohol abuse or dependence
- Typically invest considerable advance preparation for starting a fire
- Reaction to the consequences can range from indifference to satisfaction from the resulting property destruction

9.6 Pathological Gambling

9.6.1 Diagnosis

ICD-10 Diagnostic Guidelines (F63.0)

- Frequent, repeated episodes of gambling which dominate the individual's life to the detriment of social, occupational, material, and family values and commitments
- Intense urge to gamble, which is difficult to control, together with preoccupation with ideas and images of the act of gambling and the circumstances that surround the act
- Patients may put jobs at risk, acquire large debts, and lie or break the law to obtain money or evade payment of debts

Summary of DSM-IV-TR Diagnostic Guidelines (312.31)

- Persistent maladaptive gambling behavior and a preoccupation with gambling
- Gambles to escape from problems or to relieve anxiety and depression
- Gambles increasingly higher sums to achieve desired excitement
- Significant social and legal disruption including concealment and lying about gambling behavior, committing illegal acts or relying on others to fund gambling, disruption or loss of family, employment, or educational activities due to gambling
- Anxious and irritable between gambling rounds; previous attempts to quit gambling have been unsuccessful
- The behavior should not be caused by manic episode

For exact diagnostic criteria, please refer to the DSM-IV-TR.

9.6.2 Epidemiology

Approximately 1% of individuals meet criteria for pathological gambling; an estimated 3%-5% of the population are problem gamblers.

9.6.3 Etiology

Psychosocial

- Early parental loss, inappropriate parental discipline, focus on materialism in family dynamic

Neurobiological

- Dopamine and serotonin transmission under investigation

9.6.4 Course

- Waxes and wanes, but tends to be chronic
- Four phases typically characterize Pathological Gambling

Phase	Characteristics
Winning	Ends with a "big win" (eg, a year's salary)
Progressive loss	Life becomes structured around gambling with concomitant toll on finances, career, personal life
Desperate phase	Individual becomes increasingly indebted, and may become involved in underground economy
Hopeless	Arousal/excitement sustains gambling despite awareness of financial futility and odds of recovering with a "win"

9.6.5 Differential Diagnosis

- Social gambling (restricted to friends or family; predetermined acceptable losses)
- Professional gambling (limited risks; focus on discipline regarding risk management)
- Manic episode
- Antisocial personality disorder

9.6.6 Treatment

- Gamblers Anonymous
- Cognitive behavioral therapy
- Potential role for fluvoxamine, clomipramine, lithium

9.6.7 Comorbidities

- Substance abuse disorders (esp. alcohol and cocaine abuse; caffeine and nicotine dependence)
- Mood disorders (esp. major depressive disorder and bipolar disorder)
- Attention deficit hyperactivity disorder (ADHD)
- Personality disorders (narcissistic, antisocial, borderline, obsessive-compulsive traits)
- Other impulse control disorders

9.7 Trichotillomania

9.7.1 Diagnosis

ICD-10 Diagnostic Guidelines (F63.3)
- Characterized by noticeable hair loss due to a recurrent failure to resist impulses to pull out hairs
- Hair-pulling is usually preceded by mounting tension and is followed by a sense of relief or gratification
- Rule out pre-existing skin inflammation and psychosis

Summary of DSM-IV-TR Diagnostic Guidelines (312.39)
- Repeated hair pulling resulting in noticeable hair loss
- Increased sense of tension prior to the act followed by gratification and relief during and after the act
- The behavior should not be caused by other mental disorders or medical conditions and should cause significant functional impairment

For exact diagnostic criteria, please refer to the DSM-IV-TR.

9.7.2 Epidemiology

- Equally prevalent in males and females in childhood
- Females overrepresented in adulthood
- Lifetime prevalence ranges from 0.6%-3.4% in the general population
- More serious, chronic form begins in early to mid-adolescence
- Approximately 1/3 of patients with Trichotillomania chew or swallow their hair; with bezoars forming in about a 1/3 of these patients

9.7.3 Etiology

- Trichotillomania is linked to stressful situations in over a quarter of all cases
- Disturbances in mother-child relationships, fear of being left alone, recent object loss
- Substance use
- Depressive symptoms
- Genetic
  - Increased prevalence of tic disorder, impulse-control disorders and obsessive compulsive symptoms in family members

9.7.4 Course

- Onset is typically before 17 years of age
- Duration is typically greater than 1 year
- Both chronic and remitting forms occur

Onset	Prognosis
Early (<6 yrs old)	Good prognosis; readily responds to behavioral strategies
Late (>13 yrs old)	More likely to have chronic course, poorer prognosis

9.7.5 Differential Diagnosis

- Other causes of alopecia:
  - Alopecia areata, male pattern baldness, chronic discoid lupus erythematosus, lichen planopilaris, folliculitis decalvans, pseudopelade, alopecia mucinosa
- Schizophrenia (secondary to delusions or hallucinations)
- Obsessive compulsive disorder (in response to obsession or according to rigid rules)
- Stereotypic movement disorder
- Factitious disorder with predominantly physical signs and symptoms (motivated by secondary gain of sick role)
- "Habit" in children, particularly if behavior persists for less than several months

9.7.6 Treatment

- No consensus regarding treatment
- Psychiatry often works in conjunction with dermatology

Drugs

- Topical steroids
- Hydroxyzine hydrochloride
- Anxiolytic with antihistamine properties
- Antidepressants →197
- SSRIs →201
- Antipsychotics

Behavioral Interventions

- Biofeedback
- Self-monitoring
- Covert desensitization
- Habit reversal
- Behavior therapy

Psychotherapy

- Insight-oriented psychotherapy (for chronic form)
- Hypnotherapy

9.8   Impulse Control Disorder Not Otherwise Specified (NOS)

The DSM-IV-TR specifies this residual category be used for:
- Disorders of impulse control (eg, such as skin picking) that do not meet the criteria for any specific Impulse Control Disorder
- Another mental disorder with features involving impulse control (eg, substance dependence, paraphilia)

Note: Must differentiate between impulse and compulsion, both of which are associated with a preceding state of increased tension.

	Impulse	Compulsion
Associated with a resulting action/behavior	+/-	Always
Outcome	Ego-syntonic (expectation of pleasure)	Typically ego-dystonic, but exceptions exist (eg, compulsion to play videogames may be pleasurable)
Characteristics	Repetitive behaviors result in psychosocial impairments	Less risk of resulting psychosocial impairment

10 Dissociative and Somatoform Disorders

10.1 Classification

Dissociative Disorders

ICD-10 Classification of Dissociative (Conversion) Disorders (F44)	
F44.0	Dissociative amnesia
F44.1	Dissociative fugue
F44.2	Dissociative stupor
F44.3	Trance and possession disorders
F44.4	Dissociative motor disorders
F44.5	Dissociative convulsions
F44.6	Dissociative anesthesia and sensory loss
F44.7	Mixed dissociative (conversion) disorders
F44.8	Other dissociative (conversion) disorders
F44.80	Ganser's syndrome
F44.81	Multiple personality disorder
F44.82	Transient dissociative (conversion) disorders occurring in childhood and adolescence
F44.88	Other specified dissociative (conversion) disorders
F44.9	Dissociative (conversion) disorder, unspecified
DSM-IV-TR Classification of Dissociative Disorders	
300.6	Depersonalization disorder
300.12	Dissociative amnesia
300.13	Dissociative fugue
300.14	Dissociative identity disorder
300.15	Dissociative disorder NOS

Somatoform Disorders

ICD-10 Classification of Somatoform Disorders	
F45.0	Somatization disorder
F45.1	Undifferentiated somatoform disorder
F45.2	Hypochondriacal disorder
F45.3	Somatoform autonomic dysfunction
F45.30	Heart and cardiovascular system
F45.31	Upper gastrointestinal tract
F45.32	Lower gastrointestinal tract
F45.33	Respiratory system
F45.34	Genitourinary system
F45.38	Other organ or system
F45.4	Persistent somatoform pain disorder
F45.8	Other somatoform disorders
F45.9	Somatoform disorder, unspecified
DSM-IV-TR Classification of Somatoform Disorders	
300.81	Somatization disorder
300.82	Undifferentiated somatoform disorder
300.11	Conversion disorder[1]
307.80	Pain disorder, associated with psychological factors
307.89	Pain disorder, associated with both psychological factors and a general medical condition
300.7	Hypochondriasis[2]
300.7	Body dysmorphic disorder
300.82	Somatoform disorder NOS

[1]Specify type: With motor symptom or deficit/with sensory symptom or deficit/with seizures or convulsions/with mixed presentation

[2]Specify if: With poor insight

Other Disorders

ICD-10 Classification of Other Neurotic Disorders (F48.x)	
F48.0	Neurasthenia
F48.1	Depersonalization-derealization syndrome
F48.8	Other specified neurotic disorders
F48.9	Neurotic disorder, unspecified

10.2 Dissociative Disorders

10.2.1 Dissociative Amnesia (Formerly Psychogenic Amnesia)

Epidemiology
- Prevalence: Approximately 6% of the general population
- Equal incidence between males and females
- Onset difficult to assess given children's limited ability to describe subjective experience, with most reports beginning in late adolescence

Etiology
- Adverse life events such as extreme, acute trauma, profound intrapsychic conflict or emotional stress. Acute dissociative amnesia often arises out of intolerable emotions including shame, rage, guilt, or desperation
- Personal or family history of somatoform or dissociative symptoms predispose to acute amnesia development during traumatic events
- History childhood or adult abuse or trauma
- Combat exposure with a high index of intensity

Diagnosis

ICD-10 Diagnostic Guidelines (F44.0)
- Amnesia, either partial or complete, for recent events that are of a traumatic or stressful nature and is too extensive to be explained by ordinary forgetfulness (may emerge only when other informants are available)
- Absence of organic brain disorders, intoxication, or excessive fatigue
- The amnesia is usually centred on traumatic events, such as accidents or unexpected bereavements, and is usually partial and selective
- Perplexity, distress, and varying degrees of attention-seeking behavior may be evident, but calm acceptance is also sometimes striking
- Purposeless local wandering may occur; it is usually accompanied by self-neglect and rarely lasts more than a day or two

Summary of DSM-IV-TR Diagnostic Guidelines (300.12)
- One or more episodes of inability to recall important personal information, usually of a traumatic or stressful nature, that is too extensive to be explained by ordinary forgetfulness
- Disturbance is not caused by other psychiatric disorders, general medical conditions, or substance abuse
- Causes distress in important areas of functioning

For exact diagnostic criteria, please refer to the DSM-IV-TR.

Types of memory disturbances described in Dissociative Amnesia include:

Type	Nature of memory disturbance
Localized amnesia	Unable to recall events that occurred during a circumscribed time period
Selective amnesia	Able to recall some, but not all, events in a given time period
Generalized amnesia	Inability to recall one's entire life (rare)
Continuous amnesia	Inability to recall events subsequent to a specific time up to and including the present (rare)
Systematized amnesia	Memory loss for certain information categories (eg, events pertaining to an individual or one's family) (rare)

Course

Often spontaneously resolves when individual is removed from overwhelming or traumatic stressors, but the disability can extend to become a chronic generalized, continuous, or severe localized form requiring high levels of social support

Differential Diagnosis

- Ordinary forgetfulness and nonpathological amnesia (eg, childhood amnesia prior to age five)
- Posttraumatic amnesia secondary to head injury
- Seizure disorders, in particular complex partial seizure disorder
- Substance-related amnesia (eg, blackouts secondary to alcohol abuse)
- Transient global amnesia
- Acute stress disorder, posttraumatic stress disorder, and somatoform disorders
- Malingering and factitious amnesia
- Dementia, delirium and organic amnestic disorders

Treatment

- Risk management involving explicit screening for comorbid self-harm behavior or suicidal and homicidal ideation (rare)
- Cognitive therapy
- Hypnosis
- Somatic therapies
- Group psychotherapy
- Treat comorbid conditions with pharmacotherapy as appropriate

Comorbidities
- Depression +/- suicidal ideation
- Conversion or somatoform symptoms
- Depersonalization
- Derealization
- Trance states
- Spontaneous regression in age
- Ongoing anterograde dissociative amnesia

10.2.2 Dissociative Fugue

ICD-10 Diagnostic Guidelines (F44.1)

The features of **dissociative amnesia (F44.0)** plus:
- Purposeful travel beyond the usual everyday range (the differentiation between travel and wandering must be made by those with local knowledge)
- Maintenance of basic self-care (eating, washing, etc.) and simple social interaction with strangers (eg, buying food or gas, asking directions, ordering meals)

Summary of DSM-IV-TR Diagnostic Guidelines (300.13)
- Sudden and unexpected travel away from home or work with inability to recall the past
- Confusion about identity, or partial or total assumption of new identity
- Does not occur in the context of Dissociative Identity Disorder, substance abuse or other medical conditions
- Causes significant distress and functional impairment

For exact diagnostic criteria, please refer to the DSM-IV-TR.

10.2.3 Dissociative Stupor

ICD-10 Diagnostic Guidelines (F44.2)
- Stupor characterized by a profound diminution or absence of voluntary movement and normal responsiveness to external stimuli such as light, noise, and touch; total or partial absence of speech and spontaneous and purposeful movement; disturbance of consciousness, muscle tone, posture, breathing, and sometimes eye-opening and coordinated eye movements
- Absence of a physical or other psychiatric disorder that might explain the stupor
- Evidence of recent stressful events or current problems

Summary of DSM-IV-TR Diagnostic Guidelines

No equivalent diagnostic classification in the DSM-IV-TR.

10.2.4 Trance and Possession Disorders

ICD-10 Diagnostic Guidelines (F44.3)

- Temporary loss of both the sense of personal identity and full awareness of the surroundings; in some instances the individual acts as if taken over by another personality, spirit, deity, or "force"
- Attention and awareness may be limited to or concentrated upon only one or two aspects of the immediate environment, and there is often a limited but repeated set of movements, postures, and utterances
- Only unwanted, intrusive trances that are outside of cultural or religious ceremonies should be included here
- Psychosis, multiple personality disorder and intoxication should be ruled out

Summary of DSM-IV-TR Diagnostic Guidelines

No equivalent diagnostic classification in the DSM-IV-TR.

10.2.5 Dissociative Disorders of Movement and Sensation

ICD-10 Diagnostic Guidelines (F44.4–44.7)

General Guidelines

- Disorders manifest with loss of or interference with movements or sensations (usually cutaneous)
- No evidence of a physical disorder can be found to explain the symptoms despite patient's presentation with a physical disorder; symptoms can often be seen to represent the patient's concept of physical disorder, and may be at odds with physiological or anatomical principles
- Assessment of the patient's mental state and social situation usually suggests that the disability resulting from the loss of functions is helping the patient to escape from an unpleasant conflict, or to express dependency or resentment indirectly
- Although problems or conflicts may be evident to others, the patient often denies their presence and attributes any distress to the symptoms or the resulting disability
- A variable amount of attention-seeking behavior may be present in addition to a central and unvarying core of loss of movement or sensation which is not under voluntary control
- Sufficient must be known about the psychological and social setting and personal relationships of the patient to allow a convincing formulation to be made of the reasons for the appearance of the disorder
- Must rule out subtle signs of neurological conditions such as early multiple sclerosis or systemic lupus erythematosus, as well as psychiatric disorders such as schizophrenia or severe depression

ICD-10 Diagnostic Guidelines (F44.4–44.7)

Dissociative Motor Disorders (F44.4)

- Loss of ability to move the whole or a part of a limb or limbs; paralysis may be partial, with movements being weak or slow, or complete
- Various forms and variable degrees of incoordination (ataxia) may be evident, particularly in the legs, resulting in bizarre gait or inability to stand unaided (astasia-abasia)
- Possible presence of exaggerated trembling or shaking of one or more extremities or the whole body

Dissociative convulsions (F44.5)

- Dissociative convulsions (pseudoseizures) closely mimicking epileptic seizures
- Absence of serious seizure symptoms or injuries such as tongue-biting, serious bruising due to falling, and incontinence of urine
- The loss of consciousness of epileptic seizures is absent or replaced by a state of stupor or trance

Dissociative anesthesia and sensory loss (F44.6)

- Cutaneous anesthetic areas that are inconsistent with dermatomal distribution
- Differential loss between the sensory modalities that is inconsistent with neural pathways or possible neurological lesions
- Sensory loss may be accompanied by complaints of paraesthesia
- If visual disturbances are present, they are typically associate with a loss of acuity, general blurring of vision, or "tunnel vision" rather than total vision loss; patient's general mobility and motor performance are often surprisingly well-preserved

Mixed dissociative (conversion) disorders (F44.7)

- Disorders with mixed features from other dissociative disorders of movement and sensation (F44.0–F44.6)

Summary of DSM-IV-TR Diagnostic Guidelines

The DSM-IV-TR classifies many of these conditions not as Dissociative Disorders, but as **Somatoform Disorders**. Please refer to the DSM-IV-TR diagnostic guidelines summaries for somatoform disorders in the next section.

10.2.6 Conversion Disorder

ICD-10 Diagnostic Guidelines

Classified under **Dissociated Disorders of Movement and Sensation (F44.4–F44.7)** in the ICD-10 →160

Summary of DSM-IV-TR Diagnostic Guidelines (300.11)

- Motor or sensory symptoms suggestive of a neurological or medical condition that cannot be fully explained after appropriate investigation to be related to medical causes, substance use or cultural customs
- Symptoms are preceded by conflicts or other stressors
- Symptoms cause clinically significant distress and impairment in functioning

For exact diagnostic criteria, please refer to the DSM-IV-TR.

10.2.7 Dissociative Identity Disorder

ICD-10 Diagnostic Guidelines (F44.81)

Classified as **Multiple Personality Disorder** (F44.81) in the ICD-10.

- The essential feature is the apparent existence of two or more distinct personalities within an individual, with only one of them being evident at a time
- Each personality is complete, with its own memories, behavior, and preferences; these may be in marked contrast to the single premorbid personality
- One personality is usually dominant but neither has access to the memories of the other and the two are almost always unaware of each other's existence
- Change from one personality to another in the first instance is usually sudden and closely associated with traumatic events. Subsequent changes are often limited to dramatic or stressful events, or occur during sessions with a therapist that involve relaxation, hypnosis, or abreaction

Summary of DSM-IV-TR Diagnostic Guidelines (300.14)

- The presence of two or more distinct identities or personalities, at least two of which recurrently control the person's behavior
- Amnesia of important personal information that is too extensive to be explained by ordinary forgetfulness
- Not caused by intoxication or general medical conditions

For exact diagnostic criteria, please refer to the DSM-IV-TR.

10.3 Somatoform Disorders

10.3.1 Somatization Disorder

ICD-10 Diagnostic Guidelines (F45.0)

A definite diagnosis requires the presence of all of the following:

- **At least 2 years** of multiple and variable physical symptoms for which no adequate physical explanation has been found
- Persistent refusal to accept the advice or reassurance of several doctors that there is no physical explanation for the symptoms
- Some degree of impairment of social and family functioning attributable to the nature of the symptoms and resulting behavior.

Summary of DSM-IV-TR Diagnostic Guidelines (300.81)

- A history of many physical complaints beginning before age 30 years that occur over a period of several years and result in treatment being sought or significant impairment in social, occupational, or other important areas of functioning
- Symptoms include pain, GI complaints, sexual symptoms, and pseudoneurological symptoms
- Symptoms cannot be appropriately explained by a medical condition or substance use, or are disproportionate to existing medical conditions
- The symptoms are not intentionally feigned

For exact diagnostic criteria, please refer to the DSM-IV-TR.

10.3.2 Undifferentiated Somatoform Disorder

ICD-10 Diagnostic Guidelines (F45.1)

- Multiple, varying and persistent physical complaints, but the complete and typical clinical picture of somatization disorder is not fulfilled
- Compared to somatization disorder, the forceful and dramatic manner of complaint may be lacking, the complaints may be fewer in number, or the associated impairment of social and family functioning may be totally absent

Summary of DSM-IV-TR Diagnostic Guidelines (300.82)

- One or more physical complaints such as fatigue, loss of appetite, gastrointestinal or urinary complaints lasting **at least 6 months**
- Symptoms cannot be appropriately explained by a medical condition or substance use, or are disproportionate to existing medical conditions
- The symptoms cause clinically significant distress or impairment in functioning
- Symptoms are not intentionally feigned or caused by other mental disorders

For exact diagnostic criteria, please refer to the DSM-IV-TR.

10.3.3 Hypochondriacal Disorder

ICD-10 Diagnostic Guidelines (F45.2)

For a definite diagnosis, **both of the following** should be present:

- Persistent belief in the presence of at least one serious physical illness underlying the presenting symptom or symptoms, even though repeated investigations and examinations have identified no adequate physical explanation, or a persistent preoccupation with a presumed deformity or disfigurement
- Persistent refusal to accept the advice and reassurance of several different doctors that there is no physical illness or abnormality underlying the symptoms

Includes **Body Dysmorphic Disorder**

Summary of DSM-IV-TR Diagnostic Guidelines (300.7)

- Preoccupation with fears of having a serious disease based on misinterpreted symptoms despite appropriate medical evaluation and reassurance
- Symptoms last at least 6 months and cause significant distress and functional impairment
- Symptoms not better accounted by other mental disorders

For exact diagnostic criteria, please refer to the DSM-IV-TR.

10.3.4 Body Dysmorphic Disorder

ICD-10 Diagnostic Guidelines

Coded under **Hypochondriacal Disorder (F45.2)** in the ICD-10.

Summary of DSM-IV-TR Diagnostic Guidelines (300.7)

Excessive preoccupation with a slight or imagined physical defect that causes marked distress or functional impairment.

For exact diagnostic criteria, please refer to the DSM-IV-TR.

10.3.5 Pain Disorders

ICD-10 Diagnostic Guidelines (F45.4)

- The predominant complaint is of persistent, severe, and distressing pain, which cannot be explained fully by a physiological process or a physical disorder
- Pain occurs in association with emotional conflict or psychosocial problems that are sufficient to allow the conclusion that they are the main causative influences.
- Pain associated with depressive disorder or schizophrenia, or caused by muscle tensions or migraine should not be coded here

Summary of DSM-IV-TR Diagnostic Guidelines (307.8x)

- Significant pain in one or more sites causing significant distress and functional impairment
- Psychological factors play a key role in the onset, intensity and exacerbation of the pain
- The pain is not intentionally feigner or better explained by a medical condition or another mental disorder

Subtypes:

- Pain Disorder Associated With Psychological Factors (307.80)
- Pain Disorder Associated With Both Psychological Factors and a General Medical Condition (307.89)

For exact diagnostic criteria, please refer to the DSM-IV-TR.

10.3.6 Somatoform Autonomic Dysfunction

ICD-10 Diagnostic Guidelines (F45.3x)

Definite diagnosis requires **all of the following:**
- Symptoms of autonomic arousal, such as palpitations, sweating, tremor, flushing, which are persistent and troublesome
- Additional subjective symptoms referred to a specific organ or system
- Preoccupation with and distress about the possibility of a serious (but often unspecified) disorder of the stated organ or system, which does not respond to repeated explanation and reassurance by doctors
- No evidence of a significant disturbance of structure or function of the stated system or organ

Summary of DSM-IV-TR Diagnostic Guidelines

No equivalent diagnostic classification in the DSM-IV-TR.

10.4   Other Neurotic Disorder

10.4.1 Depersonalization Disorder

ICD-10 Diagnostic Guidelines (F48.1)

Classified as Depersonalization-Derealization Syndrome (F48.1) in the ICD-10. A definitive diagnosis requires the **presence of (a) and/or (b) plus (c) and (d):**
a. Depersonalization symptoms, ie, the individual feels that his or her own feelings and/or experiences are detached, distant, not his or her own, lost, etc
b. Derealization symptoms, ie, objects, people, and/or surroundings seem unreal, distant, artificial, colourless, lifeless, etc
c. Insight manifested by an acceptance that this is a subjective and spontaneous change, not imposed by outside forces or other people (ie, no psychosis)
d. A clear sensorium and absence of toxic confusional state or epilepsy.

Summary of DSM-IV-TR Diagnostic Guidelines (300.6)

- Persistent or recurrent experiences of feeling detached from one's mental processes or body, as if an outside observer
- Absence of psychosis, intact reality testing
- Does not occur in context of another psychiatric condition, intoxication or general medical condition

For exact diagnostic criteria, please refer to the DSM-IV-TR.

11 Substance Related Disorders

11.1 General Overview

11.1.1 Introduction

Approximately half of the world population uses at least one psychoactive substance. Worldwide, drug and alcohol use disorders (excluding tobacco) are the sixth leading cause of disease burden in adults.

11.1.2 Neurobiology

- Many neuronal circuits and neurotransmitters are part of the process of addiction
- In addition to dopamine, the neurotransmitters glutamate, gamma-amino-butyric acid (GABA), and opioid neuropeptides are important in substance-related disorders
- Susceptibility to addiction seems to be influenced by genetics
- The genetic contribution is determined by multiple genes and is modulated by environmental influences

11.1.3 Classification

- DSM-IV-TR defines a substance as "a drug of abuse, a medication, or a toxin" and classifies disorders attributable to substance use.

Substance Related Disorders (Using Alcohol Use As an Example)	
Substance Use Disorder	**Substance Induced Disorder**
Dependence	**Intoxication**
Maladaptive drinking leading to clinically significant impairment or distress, shown by **3+** of the following in the same 12-month period: • Drinking more or longer than intended • Persistent desire or unsuccessful efforts to cut down or stop • A great deal of time spent on drinking or getting over its effects • Important activities given up or reduced because of drinking • Continued drinking despite knowledge of a serious physical or psychological problem • Tolerance • Withdrawal, or drinking to avoid or relieve withdrawal	A person is said to suffer from alcohol intoxication when the quantity of alcohol the person consumes exceeds the individual's tolerance for alcohol and produces behavioral or physical abnormalities. In other words, the person's mental and physical abilities are impaired.
Abuse	**Withdrawal**
Not dependent, and maladaptive drinking leading to clinically significant impairment or distress, shown by **1+** of the following: • Continued use despite social/interpersonal problems • Hazardous use (eg, driving when impaired by alcohol) • Frequent drinking leading to failure to function in major roles • Legal problems	Alcohol withdrawal refers to the physiological symptoms that occur once alcohol use is stopped after heavy drinking. It may occur after a single episode of very heavy use, or after a prolonged or chronic period of use. Its symptoms are serious and can be potentially deadly (ie, delirium tremens).

- Eleven classes of substances that include the commonly recognized abusable drugs are described; other medications or toxins that could cause disorders are grouped into the class of other or unknown
- The specific substance-related disorders are the substance-induced disorders of intoxication and withdrawal and the substance use disorders of abuse and dependence

11.1.4 Approach to the Patient

A patient with a substance use disorder may present in a number of different ways:
- Mood problems, anxiety, sleep difficulties, or symptoms of another Axis I or Axis II psychiatric disorder
- All patients should be routinely and consistently screened for substance use disorders
- It is useful to begin with the CAGE-D instrument of questioning because the patient's answers to the questions can serve as a springboard into further discussion of substance use
- Inquire about all classes of substances (eg, alcohol, opioids, sedative/hypnotics, stimulants, cannabis, nicotine), including prescription medications as well as legal and illegal substances, because a patient may not regard abuse of some substances to be as significant as that of others
- General physical examination
- Laboratory studies

11.1.5 Treatment: General Principles

Withdrawal

Treatment of withdrawal is generally accomplished by one or a combination of two general methods:
- The first option is to use a cross-tolerant longer-acting medication in substitution of the drug of abuse (eg, methadone for heroin, nicotine for tobacco smoke, diazepam for alcohol). The dosage is adjusted until withdrawal symptoms are minimized, and then the medication is gradually tapered off
- The second option is non-cross-tolerant medications are used to reduce withdrawal-associated symptoms (eg, clonidine for opioid withdrawal, bupropion for nicotine withdrawal)
- Treatment of substance withdrawal alone does little to improve outcomes for patients with substance use disorders
- The time during the treatment of withdrawal should also be used to enhance motivation and initiate treatment for abuse or dependence

Substance Use Disorders

The type of treatment employed for substance abuse ideally depends on the patient's acceptance of or motivation for treatment, the severity of the patient's substance-related problems, and other, yet-to-be-identified factors

Substance Use Disorders

- The Stages of Change model by Prochaska is useful for conceptualizing a patient's motivation to address substance use problems. (Precontemplation, Contemplation, Preparation, Action and Maintenance)

Psychotherapies

- Psychosocial, psychotherapeutic, or behavioral interventions are the mainstays for recovery from substance use disorders

Goal

- The optimal goal for the individual patient with substance dependence is abstinence from all non-medically supervised substance use

11.2 Alcohol

11.2.1 Epidemiology

It is estimated that 7.6% (18.2 million) of persons age 12 years or older met the criteria for alcohol dependence or abuse.

11.2.2 Risk Factors

- Men
- Lower socioeconomic groups
- Lower education levels
- Young
- Certain professions are also associated with heavy drinking and drink-related harm
- Drinks industry workers, travelling sales associates, physicians

11.2.3 Genetics

- First degree relatives have double the risk of alcohol problems
- Children have increased risk even when adopted into families without alcohol problems
- No causative genes for alcoholism have been identified

11.2.4 Comorbidities

- Most patients with alcoholism have at least one other psychiatric disorder
- Women: Most commonly have a comorbid Axis I psychopathology

- Common comorbid condition:
  - Substance abuse (most common in men and women, more common in men)
  - Antisocial personality disorder (more common in men)

Anxiety and Depressive Disorder
- Generalized anxiety, panic attacks, and low mood are very frequently reported in alcohol abusers
- Depressive illness or anxiety disorder
- Chronic alcohol use will act as a direct depressant, and its secondary effects will further produce depressogenic life events
- Primary mood or anxiety disorder should not be treated in the presence of continuing alcohol misuse as psychological or pharmacological treatment for mood disorder is unlikely to be effective in the presence of alcohol abuse

Suicide
Schizophrenic patients are at high risk
- High rates of alcohol and substance abuse
- Increased risk of violence and delirium tremens development
- Alcohol is an easily available temporary treatment for some of the distressing symptoms of psychotic illness

Comorbid drug use[10]
- Additional drugs are used in addition to alcohol to enhance its effects or minimise its unpleasant side effects
- Comorbid drug misuse is associated with poorer outcomes
- Some comorbidity can have an iatrogenic component whereby the user begins substituting alcohol with treatment drugs (eg, benzodiazepines). This can result from inappropriate prescribing of anxiolytics, misdiagnosis of alcohol problems as anxiety disorders, and repeated unsupervised withdrawals with tablet hoarding. Aim to minimize prescription of potentially habit forming drugs

11.2.5 The Standard Drink and Blood Alcohol Content

Alcohol equivalents in different common drinks are expressed in terms of the so-called "standard drink." The content of alcohol in a standard drink varies from country to country.[a] In the US, one standard drink is equivalent to the following:[11]
- 14g of pure ethanol (approx. 0.5 ounces or 1.2 tablespoons)
- 12 ounces of beer or cooler (5% EtOH content)
- 5 ounces of wine (12% EtOH content, one fifth of a typical 750 mL wine bottle)
- 1.5 ounces of an 80 proof hard liquor

a. Other standard drinks: Australia: 10g, Austria: 6g, France: 12g, Japan:19.7g, UK: 7.9g

The blood alcohol content (BAC) is expressed in mg/dL. Using this measure, 100 mg/dL is 1 part EtOH in 1000 parts of blood, or 0.10% concentration. Impairment usually begins occurring at approx. 0.05%, depending on tolerance and other factors.

The BAC depends on the rate of EtOH absorption in the intestine and the rate of metabolism by the liver. Absorption varies markedly with food consumption (slower when consumed with food, especially fatty foods), and to a lesser degree gender. The rate of metabolism depends on race, gender, weight and other genetic factors. This rate can increase considerably over time from chronic use, due to enzyme upregulation in the liver, but in general it is roughly constant over short intervals.

The general rule of thumb is that a standard drink increases BAC by 15-20 mg/dL and takes about 1 hour to metabolize. However, this can vary markedly with the factors listed above (eg, weight, sex, genetics, tolerance, etc).

11.2.6 Prognosis [12]

Favorable prognostic signs
- Absence of pre-existing antisocial personality disorder
- Absence of other substance-related problems
- Having a job
- Close family contacts
- Absence of severe legal problems
- Compliance for the full course of the initial rehabilitation

11.2.7 Intoxication

- Impairment is dependent on the individual's tolerance, the amount and type of alcoholic beverage ingested, and the amount absorbed
- Blood alcohol level of 0.4 g/dL is associated with a 50% mortality risk in non-alcoholic persons
- In determining how quickly a blood alcohol level will decrease, a rule of thumb is that the body metabolizes approximately one drink (approximately 15 mg/dL) per hour

11.2.8 Withdrawal

General Overview

- Alcohol withdrawal
  - Begins 6-8 hours after the last drink
  - Symptoms usually resolve within 24-28 hours in mild to moderate withdrawal, but may be significantly longer (a week) in severe or complicated withdrawal (eg, DT)
- The spectrum of alcohol withdrawal symptoms is wide
- Only about 5% of individuals with alcohol dependence will develop more than mild to moderate withdrawal symptoms

Summary of DSM-IV-TR Diagnostic Guidelines for Alcohol Withdrawal

- Stopping or reducing alcohol consumption after a prolonged period of heavy use
- Symptoms including tachycardia, diaphoresis, tremors, insomnia, nausea, vomiting, illusions or hallucinations, psychomotor aggitation or instability, anxiety, or seizures developing within hours to days after alcohol cessation

For exact diagnostic criteria, please refer to the DSM-IV-TR.

Alcohol Hallucinosis

- Occurs in 3%-10% of patients with severe alcohol withdrawal
- Presents as auditory, visual, or tactile hallucinations
- Not dependent and maladaptive drinking leading to clinically significant impairment or distress, shown by 1+ of the following:
  - Continued use despite social/interpersonal problems
  - Hazardous use (eg, driving when impaired by alcohol)
  - Frequent drinking leading to failure to function in major roles
  - Legal problems

Delirium Tremens

- Agitation and tremulousness, autonomic instability, fevers, auditory and visual hallucinations, and disorientation
- Usually develops 2-4 days from the person's last drink
- The average duration is less than 1 week
- Occurs in 5% of patients admitted for alcohol withdrawal
- Medical emergency: Mortality rate can be as high at 20% without prompt and adequate treatment of the severe withdrawal

Seizures

- Occur in 5%-15% of patients
- Usually occur in the first 24 hours from last drink, but they can occur any time in the first 5 days
- Usually grand mal (generalized tonic-clonic)
- Past history of alcohol withdrawal seizures increases risk for seizures in subsequent episodes of alcohol withdrawal

11.2.9 Diagnosis

Questionnaires and Assessment

Several questionnaires are available for the detection of drinking-related problems [13]
- **CAGE**: A positive response to any of the questions on the CAGE should lead the clinician to investigate problem drinking with the patient further
  - **C**ut down: Have you ever tried to cut down on your drinking?
  - **A**nnoyed: Have you ever been annoyed by others criticizing your drinking?
  - **G**uilty: Have you ever felt guilty about your drinking?
  - **E**ye-opener: Have you ever had a drink first thing in the morning to steady your nerves or to get rid of a hangover?
- The Alcohol Use Disorders Identification Test (AUDIT) is another 10-item questionnaire used for the screening of alcohol use disorders

General Assessment
- When was the last drink?
- Do you have to drink more to get the same effect?
- Do you get shaky or nauseous when you stop drinking?
- Have you had a withdrawal seizure?
- How much time and effort do you put into obtaining alcohol?
- Has your drinking affected your ability to work, go to school, or have relationships?
- Have you suffered any legal consequences?
- Has your drinking caused any medical problems?

Differentiating Moderate Drinking from a Drinking Problem [14]

Moderate Drinking	Drinking Problem
Drinking within the recommended guidelines • Men: 2 or less/day • Women: 1 or less/day • Elderly: 1 or less/day	**Drinking above the recommended guidelines, associated with:** • Drinking to reduce depression or anxiety • Loss of interest in food • Lying/hiding drinking habits • Drinking alone • Injuring self or others while intoxicated • Were drunk more than three or four times last year • Increasing tolerance • Withdrawal symptoms: feeling irritable, resentful, unreasonable when not drinking • Experiencing medical, social, legal, or financial problems caused by drinking

Laboratory Data and Biological Markers [15]

- γ-Glutamyltransferase (GGT) has typically been recognized as a liver enzyme whose elevation may be more indicative of alcohol use
- Elevated red cell mean corpuscular volume (MCV), carbohydrate deficient transferrin (CDT) act as markers for excessive alcohol consumption. They are best used to monitor consumption in patients in follow-up
- MCV remains raised for 3–6 months due to 120 day lifespan

11.2.10 Treatment of Withdrawal

Management Strategies in Alcohol Detoxification

- Adjunctive treatment of comorbid medical problems
- Rehydration
- Correction of electrolyte abnormalities (including hypomagnesemia, hypophosphatemia, and hypokalemia)
- Nutritional deficiencies are common and oral multivitamin preparations containing folic acid are administered
- Replacement of thiamine is important to prevent Wernicke's encephalopathy; administer thiamine before giving glucose

- Benzodiazepines are the gold standard for the treatment of alcohol withdrawal
  - Fixed dosage and taper or on an as-needed basis
- Anticonvulsants can also be used in alcohol detoxification

Clinical Institute Withdrawal Assessment for Alcohol (CIWA-AR)

The Clinical Institute Withdrawal Assessment Scale for Alcohol-Revised is a short test rating the severity of alcohol withdrawal as observed by a health care professional. It is a 10-item assessment tool can be used to quantify the severity of alcohol withdrawal syndrome and to monitor and medicate patients going through withdrawal.

Areas of Assessment:
- Nausea and vomiting
- Tactile disturbances
- Tremor
- Auditory disturbances
- Agitation
- Paroxysmal sweats
- Visual disturbances
- Anxiety
- Headache, fullness in head
- Orientation and clouding of sensorium

Scoring: All categories are scored from 0-7 (except orientation and sensorium 0-4), maximum score of 67
  - Mild <10
  - Moderate 10-20
  - Severe >20

Benzodiazepines in Alcohol Withdrawal	
Withdrawal level	**Benzodiazepine Regimen**
Mild	Diazepam 5-10 mg PO prn Lorazepam 1-2 mg PO q 4-6h x 1-3 days
Moderate	Diazepam taper: • Day 1: 15-20 mg PO 4 times daily • Day 2: 10-20 mg PO 4 times daily • Day 3: 5-15 mg PO 4 times daily • Day 4: 10 mg PO 4 times daily • Day 5: 5 mg PO 4 times daily Lorazepam taper: • Days 1 & 2: 2-4 mg PO 4 times daily • Days 3 & 4: 1-2 mg PO 4 times daily • Day 5: 1 mg PO 4 times daily
Severe (DT)*	Diazepam 5-10 mg PO/IV every 5-15 minutes PRN Lorazepam 2-4 mg PO/IV every 5-15 minutes PRN Lorazepam SL 1-2 mg sublingual PRN Chlordiazepoxide 25 mg PO every hour PRN

*The IV route should be used in patients with DT or seizures. Benzodiazepine dose should be repeated PRN every 5-15 minutes with close monitoring until appropriate desired sedation is obtained (severe withdrawal could require significant doses). Suspect DT if doses > 50 mg diazepam or >10 mg lorazepam are required to control withdrawal during the first hour of treatment.

Treatment of Refractory DT
- Strongly consider admission to ICU as mechanical ventilation is likely
- Barbiturates may be added to benzodiazepine, eg, phenobarbital 130-260 mg IV every 15-20 min PRN until symptoms are controlled; propofol may also be used (intubation is often required if phenobarbital or propofol are used)
- Antipsychotics (eg, haloperidol) should not routinely be used as they lower the seizure threshold and may interfere with heat dissipation

Seizure management
- High dose IV benzodiazepines should be first line and generally resolve alcohol withdrawal seizures
- Phenobarbital may be added as specified above, but sustained anticonvulsant therapy should not be used in alcohol withdrawal therapy

ICU Admission Criteria [16]
- Age >40
- Cardiac disease (heart failure, arrhythmia, angina, myocardial ischemia, recent myocardial infarction)

- Hemodynamic instability
- Marked acid-base disturbances
- Severe electrolyte defects (hypokalemia, hypophosphatemia, hypomagnesemia, hypocalcemia)
- Respiratory insufficiency (hypoxemia, hypercapnia, severe hypocapnia, pneumonia, asthma, COPD)
- Potentially serious infections (wounds, pneumonia, trauma, urinary tract infection)
- Signs of gastrointestinal pathology (pancreatitis, GI bleeding, hepatic insufficiency, suspected peritonitis)
- Persistent hyperthermia (T >39°C [103°F])
- Evidence of rhabdomyolysis
- Renal insufficiency or increased fluid requirements
- History of prior alcohol withdrawal complications (eg, delirium tremens, alcohol withdrawal seizures)
- Need for frequent or high doses of sedatives or an intravenous infusion to control symptoms
- Withdrawal despite an elevated ethanol concentration

Relapse Prevention

- Maintenance of abstinence can be very difficult to achieve
  - Approximately 50% of alcoholic patients relapse within 3 months
- Psychosocial support is the cornerstone of achieving this goal
  - Three forms of individual behavioral treatment (cognitive-behavioral, motivational enhancement, and 12-Step facilitation) contribute to sustained abstinence and reduced drinking

There are three medications for maintenance treatment of alcohol dependence: Disulfiram, naltrexone (including its long-acting intramuscular formulation), and acamprosate

Disulfiram

- Alcohol deterrent drug works by interrupting the metabolism of alcohol
- Inhibits aldehyde dehydrogenase and blocks the breakdown of acetaldehyde to acetate
- When alcohol is consumed, the level of acetaldehyde increases, causing nausea, vomiting, and changes in blood pressure

Naltrexone

- The mechanism of action is not fully understood
- Competitive antagonist at the opioid receptor and is hypothesized to indirectly block alcohol-induced dopamine release

- Reduces the rewarding effects of alcohol and thereby reduce the craving to drink and loss of control
- Effective in increasing the percent of days abstinent, prolonging time to first heavy drinking day, and reducing amount of alcohol consumed per drinking episode
- Long-acting intramuscular formulation of naltrexone offers the benefit of once-monthly injections

Acamprosate

- Mechanism of action remains unclear
- Thought to interact with glutamate and GABA neurotransmitter systems to help restore this balance
- Assist in the maintenance of abstinence and to decrease negative symptoms associated with the acute post-withdrawal period in recently detoxified alcohol-dependent individuals

11.2.11 Complications

General

- Elevated blood pressure and increased risk of myocardial infarction
- Increased risk of cancer, particularly esophageal, head, neck, liver, stomach, colon, and lung
- Long-term alcoholism results in damage to the liver, cirrhosis and death
- Esophageal varices resulting from the long-term abuse of alcohol can also be life threatening when they rupture, leading to rapid, profuse bleeding

Wernicke's Encephalopathy and Wernicke-Korsakoff Syndrome

Wernicke's Encephalopathy

- Result of thiamine deficiency in alcoholism
- The syndrome can be precipitated by the administration of glucose to asymptomatic individuals with thiamine deficiency
- It is important to ensure that alcohol-dependent individuals receive supplemental thiamine before administration of glucose in an acute setting
- Symptoms include decreased concentration, apathy, mild agitation, and depressed mood. Confusion, amnesia, and confabulation are late signs of severe and prolonged deficit
- Also known as alcoholic encephalopathy, is of acute onset and reversible

Wernicke-Korsakoff Syndrome [17]

- Syndrome is chronic and largely (80%) irreversible
- Cranial nerve VIII impairment

Management [18]
- Wernicke's encephalopathy: Thiamine 100mg PO OD x1-2 weeks
- Korsakoff's psychosis: Thiamine 100mg PO BID/TID x3-12 months

Prognosis
Untreated, the acute phase lasts 2 weeks with 84% of cases developing features of Korsakoff psychosis.

Korsakoff Psychosis [19]
- Absence or significant impairment in the ability to lay down new memories, together with a variable length of retrograde amnesia. Working memory is unimpaired as is procedural and emotional memory
- Fetal alcohol syndrome results from a mother consuming alcohol during her pregnancy; no amount of alcohol can be considered safe during pregnancy. In this syndrome, mental retardation is common

11.3 Cannabis

11.3.1 Epidemiology
- Cannabis is the most commonly used illicit drug worldwide
- The average age of treatment admissions was about 10 years younger than for alcohol, opiates, or stimulants (mid- to late 20s versus mid- to late 30s)
- In many populations, alcohol and tobacco use precede marijuana use, which in turn precedes opioid or cocaine use
- A relationship has been shown between early, regular cannabis use and subsequent abuse of other drugs

11.3.2 Intoxication and Withdrawal
- No specific treatment is indicated for intoxication
- Cannabis withdrawal syndrome:
  - Begins 2-3 days after cessation of use
  - Mild, but the duration has been variable from 12 to 115 days
- No specific treatment is generally needed

11.3.3 Diagnosis and Treatment
- Careful history
- No medications have been shown to be useful for the treatment of dependence

11.3.4 Complications
- Increased risk of paranoia
- Growing evidence about associations between early onset of marijuana use and psychosis or schizophrenia

- Increased risk of certain cancers and pulmonary complications
- Women considering becoming pregnant or who are already so should be strongly advised not to use cannabis due to the following effects:
  - Fetal growth decreases
  - Cognitive and behavioral impairments
  - Psychiatric symptoms in the child

11.4 Stimulants

11.4.1 Epidemiology

- Stimulants include: Cocaine, amphetamine, and amphetamine-like substances
- Amphetamine-type substances come in several different forms:
  - Powdered methamphetamine hydrochloride ("speed", "meth", or "crank") can be snorted, injected, or dissolved in beverages
  - Pills can be prescription medications such as dexamphetamine or clandestinely manufactured tablets of powdered methamphetamine
  - Freebase methamphetamine (sometimes called "ice") can be vaporized in a pipe or on aluminum foil and insufflated (smoked), producing as rapid a high as with injection but without having to use needles

11.4.2 Intoxication

- Cocaine and amphetamines are both powerful CNS stimulants and have many similar symptoms that include euphoria, agitation, hypertension, and tachycarida. Amphetamines, especially methamphetamine, tends to present with more agitation, including psychosis (eg, hallucinations, delusions, violent behavior)
- The half-lives of these drugs differ significantly, approximately 40-60 minutes for cocaine and 6-12 hours for methamphetamine
- Chronic administration of either drug can induce a paranoid psychotic state
- Individuals may be at risk of acting violently in response to frightening delusions common in induced paranoia
- Amphetamine use can also result in delirium manifested by disorientation, confusion, fear, and anxiety

11.4.3 Withdrawal

- The symptoms of cocaine and amphetamine withdrawal are distinguished primarily by time course
  - Methamphetamine withdrawal may be more protracted and less abrupt than cocaine withdrawal
  - During the late withdrawal phase, a person may experience brief periods of intense, cue-induced drug craving, making the person very prone to reuse

- Although the physical symptoms of withdrawal are not typically life-threatening, the psychological symptoms can be profound and include severe depression, mental fatigue, vivid and unpleasant dreams, sleep disturbances, and psychomotor agitation or retardation

11.4.4 Treatment

- Psychosocial and behavioral approaches are the mainstays of treatment
- There are currently no medications for the treatment of cocaine- or amphetamine-dependent individuals
- Behavior therapies, including cognitive-behavioral therapy (CBT) and supportive-expressive psychotherapy, have been shown to help retain people in treatment and can lead to abstinence
- Positive contingency management procedures have also been shown to help an individual achieve initial abstinence

11.4.5 Complications

- Cocaine-related myocardial ischemia and infarction
- Chest pain is the most common symptom in cocaine users presenting to the emergency department, and therefore, individuals presenting with chest pain should be asked about cocaine use
- Acute coronary syndrome and cardiac arrhythmias are common in individuals presenting to emergency departments after the use of methamphetamine
- Methamphetamine use is also a risk factor for stroke, likely because its use can lead to elevations in blood pressure, vasculitis
- Methamphetamine, and "ice" in particular, is associated with increases in sex drive, decreases in sexual inhibition, and increases in risky behaviors (eg, reusing and sharing syringes, unprotected sex, and multiple sex partners)

11.5   Nicotine

11.5.1   Epidemiology

- Approximately 42.4% of U.S. adults have smoked cigarettes in the past, with half of these being current smokers
- Prevalence is higher among men and the poor
- Smoking rates decreases with increasing educational levels

11.5.2   Intoxication and Abuse

- Nicotine intoxication is not a recognized substance-induced disorder. This is because there are rarely prolonged maladaptive or clinically significant social sequelae
- Consequently, nicotine abuse is not a recognized substance use disorder

11.5.3 Diagnosis

• Diagnosis of nicotine dependence is made according to DSM-IV-TR criteria

Other rating scales may be useful in treating the disorder (eg, The Fagerström test for Nicotine Dependence)[20]

Fagerström Test for Nicotine Dependence	
Questions	Score
1. How soon after you wake up do you smoke your first cigarette • After 60 minutes (0 points) • 6-30 minutes (2 points) • 31-60 minutes (1 point) • Within 5 minutes (3 points)	
2. Do you find it difficult to refrain from smoking in places where it is forbidden? • No (0 points) • Yes (1 point)	
3. Which cigarette would you hate most to give up? • The first in the morning (1 point) • Any other (0 points)	
4. How many cigarettes per day do you smoke? • 10 or fewer (0 points) • 21-30 (2 points) • 11-20 (1 points) • 31 or more (3 points)	
5. Do you smoke more frequently during the first hours after awakening than during the rest of the day? • No (0 points) • Yes (1 point)	
6. Do you smoke if you are so ill that you are in bed most of the day? • No (0 points) • Yes (1 point)	
Add the scores for questions 1-6 for total score: Total score: 1-3= mild dependence; 4-6= moderate; >6= high	

11.5.4 Treatment and Withdrawal

- Treatment of nicotine dependence focuses on managing withdrawal and cravings and developing other behaviors that promote abstinence and prevent relapse
- The long-term (eg, 12-month) quit rates for a single attempt are less than 10%
- The lifetime long-term quit rate is approximately 50%

11.5.5 Complications

- Numerous adverse effects from long-term use including pulmonary disease (eg, bronchitis, COPD, emphysema), cardiovascular disease (eg, MI, stroke), and cancer (eg, lung cancer)
- Intoxication may occur with large doses (typically from combined use of anti-smoking remedies such as patches, gum and concurrent smoking) or from extensive contact with tobacco leaves (green tobacco sickness) or nicotine containing products. Symptoms include nausea, diarrhea, vomiting, headache, dizziness, weakness, palpitations, and diaphoresis
- Induction of hepatic enzymes and drug metabolism by the non-nicotine components of tobacco smoke
- Nicotine-dependent patients hospitalized on nonsmoking units who are stabilized on medications such as haloperidol, valproate, clozapine, oxazepam will experience decreased blood levels of the medications once discharged if they resume smoking

11.6 Sedatives and Hypnotics

11.6.1 Epidemiology

- 12% of individuals older than 12 years report lifetime abuse of sedative-hypnotic medications
- Benzodiazepines and others are commonly used in the setting of polysubstance abuse
  - They may enhance the "high" of other substances or may be used to help a person "come down" from the effects of stimulant drugs
  - They also can be used alone, particularly when taken in high doses. Barbiturates are more likely to be abused alone

11.6.2 Intoxication

- Signs and symptoms of intoxication are similar to those of alcohol intoxication:
  - Slurred speech, ataxia, and incoordination
  - At more severe levels of intoxication, stupor, and coma
- With the older nonbenzodiazepine agents, tolerance may develop to a drug's therapeutic effects but not to its toxicity, and a barbiturate overdose can be fatal
- An overdose on benzodiazepines usually never leads to death. However, if ingested along with alcohol, major tranquilizers, or opioids, the overdose can be fatal

11.6.3 Withdrawal

- Abrupt discontinuation in individuals who are physically dependent can lead to significant withdrawal symptoms, the most serious being death
- The withdrawal symptoms that occur with benzodiazepines, barbiturates, and nonbarbiturate/nonbenzodiazepine agents are similar to each other as well as to the withdrawal symptoms of alcohol
- Time course and intensity of withdrawal symptoms depend on the particular drug on which the individual is dependent

11.6.4 Treatment

Management of severe benzodiazepine overdose includes:
- Careful monitoring of the patient's airway, and ventilatory support
- Repeated doses of activated charcoal may be helpful in barbiturate or other nonbenzodiazepine ingestions
- Flumazenil, may be useful, but if not used carefully, the abruptly induced severe withdrawal can induce seizures in patients dependent on benzodiazepines
- There are four general strategies that can be used for the management of sedative-hypnotic withdrawal, including benzodiazepines:
  - Option 1: Gradually reduce the dosage of the sedative-hypnotic on which the patient is dependent
  - Option 2: Substitute a long-acting benzodiazepine (such as chlordiazepoxide) for the agent to which the person is dependent and then taper the substituted agent
  - Option 3: Substitute a long-acting barbiturate (usually phenobarbital) and then taper it
  - Option 4: Use valproate or carbamazepine
- The signs of toxicity are reliable and easily observable
- The average daily sedative-hypnotic dosage is calculated and then divided into three doses spread out over the day. If the patient is using more than one sedative-hypnotic, the total dosage equivalents of phenobarbital for all the substances combined are calculated
- Before each dose of phenobarbital, the patient is checked for signs of toxicity, and if any are present, the dose is withheld
- If minimal or no signs or symptoms of withdrawal occur, the phenobarbital dosage is decreased by 30 mg each day
- If objective signs of withdrawal develop, the daily dosage of phenobarbital is increased by 50%, and the patient is restabilized before continuing the withdrawal

11.7 Hallucinogens and Dissociatives

11.7.1 Common Types and Properties

Hallucinogens are drugs whose effects include altered sensory perception and reality distortion, and altered mood and thought patterns. Some of the hallucinogens have additional properties including amnesia, analgesia, anesthesia and dissociation.

Common Hallucinogenic Classes	
Class	**Prototypical Drugs and Effects**
Lysergic acid derivatives	• Include lysergic acid diethylamide (LSD) and plants such as morning glory (Ipomoea violacea, Rivea corymbosa) and Hawaiian baby woodrose (Argyreia nervosa) • LSDs effects include distorted time perception, visual illusions including vivid and distorted colors and hallucinations, euphoria and feelings of expansiveness, depersonalization, and a "blanding" of the senses (synesthesia); users remain oriented and aware these effects are caused by the drug
Mescaline and other phenylethylamines	• Include mescaline, the hallucinogen found in the peyote cactus and various phenylethylamines that include amphetamines, methamphetamines, MDMA, and so-called designer drugs (eg, Bromo, Blue Mystic) • The effects of these drugs are similar to LSD
Phenylcyclidine and ketamine	• Phenylcyclidine, known as PCP, is a noncompetitive NDMA receptor antagonist that acts as a dissociative anesthetic • Ketamine is also a noncompetitive NDMA receptor antagonist used in anesthesia • Both are characterized by their amnesic, analgesic anddissociative properties. Use of PCP can produce highly erratic, violent and bizarre behavior which combined with its analgesic properties make for a particularly dangerous combination
Psilocybin and other tryptamines	• Psilocybin is found in various mushrooms (commonly known as "shrooms") and produce effects similar to LSD • Tryptamines are found both in naturally occurring plants and synthetic street drugs and produce effects similar to LSD

Dextromethorphan	• A codeine analogue widely available in over-the-counter cough and cold preparations and used recreationally at doses 5-10 times the therapeutic dose • Reported to produce "out of body" dream-like states
Salvia divinorum	• A perennial herb in the mint family that is gaining popularity among teens and young adults because of easy availability on the Internet • Active ingredient is salvinorin A, a kappa opioid agonist • Produces sensory distortions (eg, synesthesia), and users report a sense of calm, elevated mood and introspection

Common Names and Classification of Hallucinogens		
Common Name	Active Ingredient	Drug Class
2CB, Bromo, Nexus	4-bromo-2,5-dimethoxyphenethylamine	Phenylethylamine
2CT-7, Blue Mystic	2,5-dimethoxy-4-N-propylthiophethylamine	Phenylethylamine
AMT	a-methyltryptamine	Indolealkylamine (tryptamine)
DMT, Ayahuasca	Dimethyltryptamine	Indolealkylamine (tryptamine)
DXM	Dextromethorphan	Arylcyclohexylamine (piperidine)
Foxy Methoxy	5-MeO-DIPT (5-methoxydimethyl tryptamine)	Indolealkylamine (tryptamine)
Hawaiian baby woodrose (Argyreia nervosa)	Ergine	Lysergamide
Ibogaine	12-methoxybogamine	Indolealkylamine (tryptamine)
K, Special K, Super K, KitKat, Ket, Vitamin K	Ketamine	Arylcyclohexylamine (piperidine)
LSD	D-lysergic acid diethylamide	Lysergamide
Mescaline, peyote	3,4,5-trimethoxy-phenethylamine	Phenylethylamine
Morning glory (Ipomoea violacea)	Lysergic acid hydroxyethylamide	Lysergamide

Common Name (cont.)	Active Ingredient	Drug Class
PCP, Angel dust	Phencyclidine	Arylcyclohexylamine (piperidine)
Magic mushrooms, shrooms	Psilocin (N,N-dimethyl-4-phosphoryloxytryptamine)	Indolealkylamine (tryptamine)
Salvia divinorum	Salvinorin A	Diterpene alkaloid

11.7.2 Epidemiology

- LSD is by far the most commonly used hallucinogen, popular in the club culture, and used by over 1 million persons in the US alone
- Mescaline is commonly used in the form of dried peyote cactus buttons that are ingested by people in certain cultures as part of religious and spiritual rituals. In the US, it may be used legally by members of the Native American Church, otherwise it is a controlled substance
- Designer phenylethylamines are popular club drugs and widely used recreationally by young adults
- Psilocybin use in the form of dried "magic mushrooms" is quite common for recreational or spiritual reasons

11.7.3 Intoxication

LSD

- Interferes with serotonin neurotransporters
- Induces euphoria in addition to delusions and visual hallucinations
- "Bad trips" can be marked by feelings of intense hallucinations, disorientation, dysphoria, and overwhelming feelings of dread and panic
- Physical effects include increased body temperature, sympathetic activation (tachycardia, hypertension, mydriasis, piloerection and diaphoresis), sleeplessness, and loss of appetite

Mescaline and other phenylethylamines

- Similar to LSD with lesser sympathetic activation
- Effects of designer street phenylethylamines are less known, but deaths have been reported with some of them

PCP and ketamine

- PCP intoxication causes severe agitation, disorientation, violent behavior, auditory hallucinations, nystagmus (vertical, horizontal and rotatory), and even catatonic stupor at high doses. Usual duration of action is 4-6 hours. Coma lasting several days may occur after severe intoxication
- PCP produces amnesia and analgesia making its users not only potentially unpredictable and violent, but also insensitive to pain, a very dangerous combination. Death often occurs from trauma suffered during intoxication

- The agitation and psychiatric disturbances caused by ketamine intoxication are much less common and severe than PCP
- Ketamine can produce depressed mental status, ataxia, and nystagmus. Massive ketamine overdoses can produce respiratory depression or apnea

Psilocybin and other tryptamines
- Neuropsychiatric effects are similar to LSD
- May cause nausea, vomiting, and diarrhea
- Tryptamines are structurally related to serotonin and may therefore produce serotonin syndrome

Dextromethorphan
- High doses can produce hallucinations, anticholinergic delirium, and coma
- Common effects including tachycardia, hypertension, lethargy, mydriasis, agitation and vomiting

Salvia divinorum
- Mild sympathomimetic symptoms
- No cases of severe toxicity or deaths have been reported

11.7.4 Withdrawal

- Hallucinogen withdrawal is not a recognized disorder
- Withdrawal symptoms of minimal clinical significance (including fatigue, irritability, and anhedonia) are reported by approximately 10% of hallucinogen users
- Although there is not a specifically defined PCP withdrawal syndrome, 25% of heavy PCP users report withdrawal symptoms of depression, anxiety, irritability, hypersomnolence, diaphoresis and tremors

11.7.5 Treatment

- Providing reassurance, support, and a calm, quiet environment are the mainstays of treatment for most cases of hallucinogen intoxication
- PCP intoxication may require more aggressive treatment due to its severe psychiatric and physiologic effects at high doses. Objects that can cause harm to patient or others should be removed from surroundings, sedatives are often required, neuroleptics may be warranted for severe psychosis. Restraints should be avoided due to risk of rhabdomyolysis
- For those individuals with extreme feelings of panic or fear, the use of a benzodiazepine may be warranted
- Neuroleptic use may be warranted for severe agitation with persistent symptoms of psychosis. Haloperidol 2-5 mg IV may be titrated to effect in severe cases
- Cases of severe toxicity causing hyperthermia, sympathetic overdrive and instability, severe agitation or other toxic effects require hospitalization and emergent care

- GI decontamination is generally not recommended in the majority of cases unless large quantities were ingested and patient presents within 1 hour of ingestion; urinary acidification is also not recommended

11.7.6 Complications

- Complications from severe hyperthermia may include rhabdomyolysis, renal failure, hepatic injury, disseminated intravascular coagulation, and multiorgan failure. Restraints should be avoided when there is a high risk of rhabdomyolysis (eg, severe PCP intoxication)
- Serotonin syndrome (triad of altered mental status, neuromuscular abnormalities, and autonomic hyperactivity) is associated with certain hallucinogens including LSD, MDMA, and Foxy Methoxy (designer tryptamine)
- Severe psychological and physiological disturbances, including coma, can occur with severe PCP intoxication
- Hallucinogen persisting perception disorder, or "flashbacks"
  - Mechanism underlying flashbacks is not clearly understood, but they have reportedly been precipitated by SSRIs
  - Flashbacks are spontaneous experiences of the same effects that occurred while a person was intoxicated with a hallucinogen in the past. Flashbacks are typically not distressing, but occasionally can produce so-called hallucinogen persisting perception disorder (HPPD) in which patients re-experience distressing and intrusive symptoms that affect daily functioning

11.8 Club Drugs

11.8.1 Epidemiology

- Drugs frequently used in all-night parties, "raves," dance clubs, and bars
- Drugs that are used in these settings include marijuana, cocaine, Methylenedioxymethamphetamine (MDMA), gamma-hydroxybutyrate (GHB), LSD, methamphetamine, flunitrazepam (Rohypnol), and ketamine
- MDMA, frequently called "Ecstasy" but also referred to as "X," "XTC," "Adam," "Clarity," and "Lover's Speed," is probably the most popular club drug used today
- GHB, also know as "G," Liquid X," "Easy Lay," and "Grievous Bodily Harm,"

11.8.2 Intoxication

Gamma-hydroxybutyrate (GHB)

- Prepared in a liquid formulation that is colorless and odorless
- Bitter and easy to disguise in drinks ingestion results in a "dreamy" stupor and amnesia
- Because of these features, GHB has been used to incapacitate victims for sexual assault (the date-rape drug)

Methylenedioxymethamphetamine (MDMA)
- Most commonly taken in tablet form
- Effects are similar to both an amphetamine and a hallucinogen
- Users of MDMA report enhanced sensations and mood, increased energy, and a strong sense of relatedness to others
- Use also results in elevations of heart rate and blood pressure as well as dilated pupils

11.8.3 Withdrawal

GHB withdrawal
Insomnia, anxiety, tremor, and intense craving
Acute symptoms usually resolve in 3-12 days

MDMA withdrawal
Fatigue, dysphoria, depression, loss of appetite and trouble concentrating

11.8.4 Treatment and Complications

Gamma-hydroxybutyrate (GBH)
- Management is largely supportive, with close monitoring
- Numerous reports in the literature of overdose with GHB leading to coma, respiratory depression, and death

Methylenedioxymethamphetamine (MDMA)
- Dehydration is a very serious concern because the drug appears to depress the sense of thirst
- Dysregulation of body temperature in addition to the high environmental temperatures at raves and increased muscular exertion from prolonged periods of dancing, has resulted in severe dehydration and rhabdomyolysis
- In addition, deaths involving MDMA use have also been related to cardiac arrhythmias, hypertensive crises, and acute renal failure
- Treatment involves rapid rehydration and core cooling
- Lorazepam may be used for agitation, panic, and seizures
- Long-term use of MDMA can result in problems with memory and mood

11.9   Inhalants

11.9.1 Epidemiology

- Often entry-point hallucinogens among young children and adolescents due to wide availability in aerosols, glues, markers, and other products
- The National Institute on Drug Abuse has specified four categories: volatile solvents, nitrites, gases, and aerosols
  - Examples: Sniffing glue, inhaling paints or sprays, and breathing contents of aerosol spray cans

11.9.2 Intoxication and Withdrawal

- Produce a rapid high that users report as similar to alcohol intoxication
- When the amount inhaled is large enough, nearly all solvents and gases produce anesthesia, a loss of sensation, and even unconsciousness
- There is no clearly documented withdrawal syndrome from inhalant use

11.9.3 Treatment and Complications

- Skin damage (burns and dermatitis)
- Cardiovascular complications:
  - Arrhythmias, myocardial ischemia from hypoxia, myocardial fibrosis, and ventricular fibrillation
- Pulmonary effects:
  - Coughing and wheezing to dyspnea, emphysema, and pneumonia
- Liver toxicity

Complications

- Metabolic acidosis or alkalosis
- Acute renal failure
- Bone marrow suppression leading to anemia and leukemia

Treatment

- Treatment is supportive and addresses the acute medical complications resulting from inhalant use
- Neurotoxicity and neuropsychiatric complications are the most common reported consequences of inhalant use
- Neurological damage:
  - Ataxia, peripheral and sensorimotor neuropathy, speech problems, and tremor
- Psychiatric symptoms resulting from inhalant use include:
  - Apathy, delirium, dementia, depression, inattention, insomnia, memory loss, and psychosis

11.10 Anabolic Androgenic Steroids

11.10.1 Epidemiology

- Category includes testosterone and its synthetic derivatives
- Abused by athletes and bodybuilders due to the effects of enhancing endurance and performance
- Also abused among male adolescents and young adults to gain muscle mass and lose fat
- The drugs can be injected, taken orally, or used transdermally

11.10.2 Intoxication

- Users report feeling good about themselves and a sense of euphoria
- AASs can produce hypomania or mania
- Extreme mood swings, irritability, aggression, and violent behavior can also result from AAS abuse
- Paranoid jealousy, extreme irritability, delusions, and impaired judgment stemming from feelings of invincibility

11.10.3 Withdrawal

- Low mood, fatigue, restlessness, anorexia, insomnia, decreased libido, and craving for steroids
- Symptoms usually resolve in several weeks, although some persons may develop more persistent symptoms of depression that may respond to treatment with SSRIs

11.10.4 Treatment

- Users rarely seek treatment
- Users may view their use as part of healthy activity when combined with a strenuous exercise regimen and otherwise healthy lifestyle
- Users can be different from other substance abusers in that the desired reward of AASs is not intoxication or a psychoactive effect but a future reward of a more muscular body or athletic success
- Motivational issues are different, as are issues regarding relapse to use

11.10.5 Complications

Major Complications:
- Liver tumors and cancer, jaundice, fluid retention, hypertension, increases in low-density lipoproteins, and decreases in high-density lipoproteins
- Kidney tumors, severe acne, and tremulousness are also potential sequelae
- Men: Include testicular atrophy, reduced sperm count, infertility, hair loss, gynecomastia, and increased risk for prostate cancer
- Women: Hirsutism may occur, including development of facial hair and male-pattern hair loss, menstrual irregularity and/or amenorrhea, clitoral enlargement, and deepening of the voice
- Adolescents: May cause premature skeletal maturation (resulting in shorter stature if they use AASs prior to the adolescent growth spurt) and accelerated pubertal changes

Progression from AAS use to other substances of abuse:
- There is a progression in AAS users to opioid dependence

11.11 Opioids

11.11.1 Epidemiology [21]

- The 2004 National Survey on Drug Use and Health estimated that:
  - 118,000 persons had used heroin for the first time within the past 12 months
  - 2.8 million persons used an illicit drug for the first time within the past 12 months, the majority of whom used a prescription opioid pain medication
- In the 2004 Monitoring the Future survey of eighth, tenth, and twelfth graders:
  - 9.3% of seniors reported using hydrocodone without a prescription in the past year, and 5% reported using oxycodone

11.11.2 Intoxication

- Opioid intoxication produces an intensely euphoric feeling often described as a "rush"
- Onset, duration, and intensity of the rush are dependent on the potency of the specific opioid use, its amount, and the route of administration (oral ingestion, inhalation, or intravenous injection)
- The classic signs of opioid intoxication include decreased mental status, decreased respiratory rate and tidal volume, decreased bowel sounds (constipation), and miotic (constricted) pupils. Effects can last for the several hours
- Overdose is life-threatening
  - Fatal respiratory depression can occur due to direct suppression of respiratory centers in the midbrain and medulla
  - Obtaining a urine drug screen can be crucial to identify not only the presence of an opioid but also that of other unsuspected drugs
  - Benzodiazepines are frequently abused with opioids, and when detected, the benzodiazepine component of the overdose can be reversed with flumazenil
  - Treatment of an opioid overdose includes general supportive management in addition to the use of naloxone, a pure opioid antagonist that can reverse the central nervous system effects of opioid intoxication and overdose

11.11.3 Withdrawal

- Repeated use of opioids creates tolerance that predispose the user towards withdrawal
- Symptoms of opioid withdrawal include:
  - Dysphoria and restlessness
  - Rhinorrhea and lacrimation
  - Myalgias and arthralgias
  - Nausea, vomiting, abdominal cramping, and diarrhea
- Timing of the withdrawal is dependent on the type of opioid used

- Administration of naloxone can produce immediate and intense withdrawal symptoms including rapid catecholamine surges and hemodynamic instability that is poorly tolerated by some patients; exercise care in naloxone administration and titrate dose to effect
- Cessation of chronic heroin use: Withdrawal symptoms begin about 8-12 hours after the last dose, peak between 36 and 72 hours, and subside over about 5 days
- Methadone: Has a much longer half-life than heroin, the peak of the withdrawal syndrome is usually between days 4 and 6, with acute symptoms persisting for 14-21 days
- Any opioid: After acute withdrawal symptoms have subsided, a protracted abstinence syndrome, including disturbances of mood and sleep, can persist for 6-8 months

11.11.4 Treatment

- Management of acute opioid withdrawal involves a combination of general supportive measures in combination with pharmacotherapy
- Option 1: Convert the patient to an equivalent dose of a longer-acting opioid and gradually taper the dose to minimize withdrawal
  - Methadone and buprenorphine are frequently used
  - In the inpatient setting, the taper is generally completed in 5-7 days, but it may need to be significantly extended in the outpatient setting to decrease the likelihood of dropout and relapse
- Option 2: Use of a clonidine (an alpha-2 adrenergic agonist) taper for amelioration of tremor, diaphoresis, and agitation
  - For expedited treatment of the withdrawal, an opioid antagonist, such as naltrexone, can be administered in conjunction with clonidine
  - Expedited withdrawal may be advantageous when a patient is withdrawing from a longer-acting agent such as methadone and would otherwise be facing a longer withdrawal treatment
  - The symptoms of expedited withdrawal may be more severe initially, so frequent patient monitoring and proactive use of adjunctive medications are essential
- With all protocols, adjuvant medications may be used:
  - Nonsteroidal anti-inflammatory for myalgias
  - Benzodiazepines or other hypnotics for short-term management of insomnia
  - Cyclobenzaprine (a muscle relaxant) can be used to treat muscle cramps
  - Dicyclomine (an anticholinergic used to reduce the contraction of muscles in the intestine) is used to treat the gastrointestinal symptoms that occur in acute withdrawal
  - Complications can include flash pulmonary edema, prolonged withdrawal, drug toxicity, rupture of varices, and aspiration pneumonia

- Maintenance treatment with agonist therapy provides relief from opioid withdrawal symptoms and thereby allows psychosocial stabilization
  - Methadone has long been considered the gold standard treatment for maintenance treatment
  - Buprenorphine is approved for detoxification and maintenance treatment of opioid dependence
- Potential advantages of buprenorphine over methadone include a longer half-life, which decreases the frequency of clinic visits, and a high safety profile with less risk of respiratory depression in overdose

11.11.5 Complications

In addition to the risk of overdose, medical comorbidities may be consequential:
- Risk of transmission of HIV, particularly in intravenous opioid users
- Hepatitis C virus
- Decreased immune function
- Hyperalgesia
- Bacterial infections (particularly with intravenous drug use), including abscesses and cellulitis of the skin
- Endocarditis with intravenous drug use is another serious concern. More than 50% of these cases will be right-sided, most often involving the tricuspid valve. Sequelae of right-sided endocarditis will often involve the lungs

11.11.6 Pregnancy Related Issues

- Opioid abuse carries an increased risk of miscarriage and premature birth
- Very high rate of relapse after detoxification, and risk of cycling between intoxication and withdrawal can be very dangerous to the fetus
- Methadone maintenance has generally been accepted as the standard approach for pregnant women
- Buprenorphine maintenance is also increasingly being used in pregnant opioid-dependent women

11.12 Polysubstance Abuse

- Polysubstance use is common
- If undetected, polysubstance use can complicate the treatment of intoxication and withdrawal
- Example: A patient in alcohol withdrawal requiring higher doses of diazepam and the syndrome continuing for 2 weeks due to concurrent, undetected benzodiazepine withdrawal
- Associated with poorer outcome and greater morbidity and mortality
- All substances must be addressed during treatment for the dependence, and the patient may have different levels of motivation for recovery from different substances

List of references

10 Oxford Michael.G. Gelder, Philip Cowen, Paul Harrison. Oxford University Press 2006
11 The United States National Institute on Alcohol Abuse and Alcoholism and the National Institute of Health
12 Comprehensive textbook of psychiatry, pg. 87
13 Babor TF, Higgins-Biddle JC, Saunders J, et al.: AUDIT, the Alcohol Use Disorders Identification Test, 2nd Edition. Geneva, Switzerland, World Health Organization, 2001; Available at: http://whqlibdoc.who.int/hq/2001/WHO_MSD_MSB_01.6a.pdf
14 Source: Toronto Notes 2010 PS20
15 Oxford Texbook of Psychiatry
16 Carlson, RW, Keske, B, Cortez, D, J Crit Illness 1998; 13:311.
17 Comprehensive textbook of psychiatry, pg. 88
18 Toronto Notes 2010, PS21
19 Oxford Textbook of Psychiatry.530-531
20 Heatherton T, Kozlowski L, Frecker R, Fagerström K. The fagerström test for nicotine dependance: A revision of the fagerström tolerance questionnaire. British J adict 1991 8b:1119-27s
21 Substance Abuse and Mental Health Services Administration 2005 Kaplan and Saddocks Comprehensive Textbook of Psychiatry

12 Drugs

12.1 Antidepressants
12.1.1 Serotonin-Norepinephrine Reuptake Inhibitors (SNRI) – Tricyclics, Tertiary Amines

MA: Inhibit reuptake of serotonin/norepinephrine into presynaptic vesicles (primarily serotonin); **AE** (SNRIs): Dry mouth, acute glaucoma, constipation, micturition disturbances, hypotension, arrhythmia, cardiomyopathy, dizziness, headache, restlessness, insomnia, confusion; **AE** (amitriptyline): Drowsiness, CVS effects, seizures, hypotension, anticholinergic effects; **AE** (clomipramine): Anticholinergic effects, somnolence, tremor, weight ↑; **AE** (doxepin): Drowsiness, CVS effects, seizures, anticholinergic effects; **AE** (imipramine): Anticholinergic effects, seizures, weight ↑, confusion, CVS effects; **AE** (trimipramine): Sedation, anticholinergic effects, weight ↑, seizures, CVS effects; **CI** (SNRIs): Glaucoma, AV block III°, combination with MAO inhibitors or Tryptophan, hypersensitivity to product ingredients/TCAs, recovery period after MI

Amitriptyline	EHL 15h (range 9-25h), Q0 1.0, PRC D/C, Lact ?
Generics Tab 10mg, 25mg, 50mg, 75mg, 100mg, 150mg	**Depression: Outpatient:** Ini 75mg/d PO (in div doses), gradually incr prn to max 150mg/d; **inpatient:** Ini 100mg/d PO in div doses, gradually incr prn to 200-300mg/d prn; IM: Ini 80-120mg IM in 4 div doses; DARF: Not req, see Prod Info

Clomipramine	EHL 19-37h (mean 32h), Q0 1.0, PRC C, Lact +
Anafranil Cap 25mg, 50mg, 75mg **Generics** Cap 25mg, 50mg, 75mg	**Obsessive compulsive DO:** Ini 25mg/d PO, gradually incr over 2wk to 100mg/d, then gradually incr prn to max 250mg/d; **CH >10 y w/ OCD:** Ini 25mg/d PO, gradual incr over 2wk prn to max 3mg/kg/d or 100mg/d, then incr prn to max 3mg/kg/d or 200mg/d

Doxepin	EHL 16.8h (range 8-25h), Q0 1.0, PRC C, Lact -
Sinequan Cap 10, 25, 50, 75, 100, 150mg, Conc (oral) 10mg/ml **Silenor** Tab 3mg, 6mg **Generics** Cap 10, 25, 50, 75, 100, 150mg, Conc (oral) 10mg/ml	**Depression:** Individualized doses, gradually incr to 75-150mg/d (outpatients) or 150-300mg/d (inpatients); DARF: Probably not req, see Prod Info; **insomnia:** 6mg PO qhs; ini 3mg in elderly pts.

Imipramine	EHL 6-18h, Q0 1.0 (1.0), PRC D, Lact ?
Tofranil Tab 10mg, 25mg, 50mg **Generics** Tab 10mg, 25mg, 50mg Conc (oral) 25mg/ml	**Depression:** Inpatients: Ini 100mg/d in div doses, gradually incr to 200mg/d prn, further incr prn after 2wk up to 250-300mg/d; outpatients: Ini 75mg/d (qd or in div doses) incr prn to max 150-200mg/d; DARF: Not req

Imipramine pamoate	EHL 11-25h, Q0 1.0 (1.0), PRC D, Lact ?
Tofranil-PM Cap 75mg, 100mg, 125mg, 150mg	**Depression:** Ini 25-75mg PO qhs, incr q3-4d by 25-50mg/d to 150-300mg/d, max 300mg/d, 100mg/d in elderly patients **chronic pain:** Ini 0.2-0.4mg/kg PO qhs, incr 50% q2-3d prn up to 3mg/kg, max 300mg/d, 100mg in elderly patients; DARF: not req

Trimipramine	EHL 23h, Q0 0.9, PRC C, Lact ?
Surmontil Cap 25mg, 50mg, 100mg	**Depression:** Outpatients: Ini 75mg/d PO in div doses, maint 50-150mg/d, max 200mg/d; inpatients: Ini 100mg/d in div doses, prn gradually incr to 200mg/d, max 250-300mg/d; adolescents: Ini 50mg/d, max 100mg/d

12.1.2 SNRI – Tricyclics, Secondary Amines

MA: Inhibit reuptake of serotonin and norepinephrine, primarily norepinephrine
Note: May cause less anticholinergic side effects than tertiary amines. Orthostatic hypotension, arrythmias. Don't use with MAOIs; **AE/CI** (SNRIs): See also SNRIs – tricyclics – tertiary amines →197; **AE** (desipramine): N/V, CVS + anticholinergic effects, sedation, seizures; **AE** (nortriptyline): Sedation, CVS + anticholinergic effects, weight gain, seizures
AE (protriptyline): CVS + anticholinergic effects, restlessness, weight gain, seizures;
CI (desipramine, nortriptyline): Concomitant use of MAO inhibitors, recovery following MI, hypersensitivity to product ingredients or TCAs; **CI** (protriptyline; additional): Administration with cisapride

Desipramine	EHL 14.3-24.7h (average 17.1h), Q0 1.0, PRC C, Lact ?
Norpramin Tab 10mg, 25mg, 50mg, 75mg, 100mg, 150mg **Generics** Tab 10mg, 25mg, 50mg, 75mg, 100mg, 150mg	**Depression:** Ini 25-75mg PO qam, maint 100-200mg qd or div, max. 300mg/d; adolescents: 25-100mg/d, max 150mg/d; DARF: See Prod Info

Nortriptyline	EHL 15-39h, Q0 1.0, PRC D, Lact ?
Aventyl HCT *Sol (oral) 10mg/5ml* **Pamelor** *Cap 10mg, 25mg, 50mg, 75mg,* *Sol (oral) 10mg/5ml* **Generics** *Cap 10mg, 25mg, 50mg, 75mg,* *Sol (oral) 10mg/5ml*	**Depression:** Ini 25-50mg PO qhs, maint 50-150mg/d (qd or div); max 150mg/d; adolescents: 30-50mg/d; DARF: Not req

Protriptyline	EHL 54-198h, PRC C, Lact ?
Vivactil *Tab 5mg, 10mg*	**Depression:** Ini 15-40mg/d PO, div tid-qid, incr prn to a max of 60mg/d

12.1.3 SNRI - Tricyclics/Polycyclics, 2nd Generation

MA: Inhibit reuptake of serotonin and norepinephrine, primarily norepinephrine
EF: Antidepressant, psychomotor sedation, anxiolytic; **AE/CI:** See also SNRIs - tricyclics - tertiary amines →197; **AE** (amoxapine): Dizziness/drowsiness, anticholinergic effects, seizures, extrapyramidal effects, CVS effects; **AE** (maprotiline): Vertigo, blurred vision, seizures, drowsiness, urinary retention; **CI** (amoxapine, maprotiline): Hypersensitivity to product ingredients, MAO inhibitors concurrently or within 2wk of therapy, MI (during acute recovery period)

Amoxapine	EHL 8h, PRC C, Lact ?
Generics *Tab 25mg, 50mg, 100mg, 150mg*	**Depression:** Ini 25-50mg PO bid-tid, maint 120-300mg/d, max 400mg/d

Maprotiline	EHL 27-58h (mean 43h), Q0 1.0, PRC B, Lact ?
Generics *Tab 25mg, 50mg, 75mg*	**Depression:** Ini 25-75mg PO qd x 2wk, (100-150mg PO qd in severe cases), incr prn by 25mg q2wk, maint 75-150mg/d, max 225mg/d; DARF: not req

12.1.4 SNRI - Non-Tricyclic

MA: Inhibit reuptake of serotonin and norepinephrine
Note: Decrease dose in renal or hepatic impairment. Monitor for increases in BP;
Don't use with MAOIs, caution with cimetidine and haloperidol; **AE** (desvenlafaxine): Dizziness, fatigue, headache, nausea, decreased apetite, dry mouth, diarrhea, constipation, interstitial lung desease, eosinophilic pneumonia, hyperhidrosis;
AE (milnacipran): N/V, headache, constipation, dizziness, insomnia, hot flush, hyperhidrosis, palpitations, increased heart rate, dry mouth, hypertension
AE (venlafaxine): Nausea, anorexia, sedation, dizziness; **CI** (desvenlafaxine): Hypersensitivity to d., concomitant use of MAOI;
CI (milnacipran): Concomitant use of MAOI, uncontrolled narrow-angle glaucoma
CI (venlafaxine): Hypersens. to venlafaxine hydrochloride, concomitant use of MAOI

Desvenlafaxine	EHL 11h, PRC C, Lact ?
Pristiq *Tab 50mg, 100mg*	**Depression:** Ini 50mg PO qd, max 400mg/d; DARF: GFR (ml/min) 30-50: max 50mg/d; <30: Max 50 mg qod

Milnacipran	EHL 6-8h, PRC C, Lact ?
Savella *Tab 12.5mg, 25mg, 50mg, 100mg*	**Fibromyalgia:** Ini12.5mg PO qd x1d, then 12.5mg bid x2d, then 25mg bid x4d, then 50mg bid; max 200mg/d; DARF: GFR (ml/min) 5-29: maint. dose 50%, max 100mg/d; <5: not recommended

Venlafaxine	EHL 5h, Q0 0.45 (0.5), PRC C, Lact ?
Effexor *Tab 25mg, 37.5mg, 50mg, 75mg, 100mg* Effexor XR *Cap ext.rel. 37.5mg, 75mg, 150mg* Generics *Tab 25mg, 37.5mg, 50mg, 75mg, 100mg; Tab ext.rel. 37.5mg, 75mg, 150mg, 225mg*	**Depression:** Ini 75mg/d PO div bid-tid (Effexor), incr by 75mg/d q 4d, max 375mg/d (in div doses); ext.rel.: ini 37.5-75mg PO qd, incr by 75mg/d q 4d, max 225mg/d; **generalized anxiety DO:** Ini 37.5-75mg PO qd (ext. rel.), incr prn by 75mg/d q 4d, max 225mg/d; **panic DO:** 37.5mg PO qd for 7d, then incr to 75mg/d, may increase prn qwk by 75mg, max 225mg/d; DARF: GFR (ml/min) 10-70: 50%-75%, <10, hemodialysis: 50%; see Prod Info

12.1.5   Norepinephrine–Dopamine Reuptake Inhibitors (NDRI)

MA: Inhibits reuptake of norepinephrine, some dopamine
AE: N/V, seizures/tremors, agitation, insomnia, hypersensitivity reactions
CI: Seizures, bulimia, anorexia, concomitant MAO inhibitors, hypersensitivity to bupropion products, concomitant use of other bupropion products

Bupropion	EHL 14h (chronic dosing: 21h), Q0 >0.8, PRC B, Lact ?
Wellbutrin *Tab 75mg, 100mg* Wellbutrin SR *Tab ext.rel. 50mg, 100mg, 150mg, 200mg* Wellbutrin XL *Tab ext.rel. 150mg, 300mg* Generics *Tab 75mg, 100mg; Tab ext. rel 100mg, 150mg, 200mg*	**Depression:** Ini 100mg PO bid, after 3d incr to 300mg/d (div tid) prn; max 150mg/dose, 450mg/d; ext. rel.: Ini 150mg PO qam, incr to 150mg bid as early as day 4; max 400mg/d div bid; **seasonal affective DO:** Ini 150mg ext.rel qam, incr to 300mg/d after 7d x 4-6mo/y; **smoking cessation** →215 DARF: Is req, see Prod Info

12.1.6 Monoamine Oxidase Inhibitors (MAOI)

MA (tranylcypromine): Irreversible inhibition of MAO type A and B ⇒ oxidative break-down ↓ ⇒ synaptic conc of epinephrine, noradrenaline, serotonin ↑
EF: Antidepressant, mainly psychomotor activation; **AE** (MAOIs): Sudden changes of BP, insomnia, restlessness, dizziness, sexual dysfunction; **CI** (MAOIs): Combination with: Other antidepressants, pethidine (= meperidine), levodopa, severe hepatic dysfunction, severe HTN, acute delirium

Isocarboxazid	EHL no data, PRC C, Lact ?
Marplan *Tab 10mg*	**Depression:** Ini10mg/d PO bid, maint 10–40mg/d, max 60mg/d div bid-qid, caution with doses over 40mg/d

Phenelzine	EHL no data, PRC C, Lact ?
Nardil *Tab 15mg*	**Depression:** Ini 15mg/d PO tid, usual effective dose 45–90mg/d in div doses DARF: not req

Tranylcypromine	EHL 1.5–3.5h, Q0 0.95, PRC C, Lact ?
Parnate *Tab 10mg*	**Depression:** Ini 10mg/d PO, incr prn by 10mg/d at 1–3wk intervals, maint 30mg/d in div doses, max 60mg/d

12.1.7 Selective Serotonin Reuptake Inhibitors (SSRI)

MA: Selective inhibition of serotonin reuptake ⇒ serotonin levels in synaptic cleft ↑
EF: Antidepressant, psychomotor activation
AE (SSRIs): Sleeplessness, agitation, somnolence, headache, N/V, diarrhea, arrhythmias, ejaculation disturbances
AE (citalopram): Nausea, dry mouth, sweating, somnolence, ejaculation DO
AE (fluoxetine): Insomnia, asthenia, tremor, headache, GI complaints
AE (fluvoxamine): Somnolence, headache, agitation, N/V, insomnia
AE (paroxetine): Headache, sedation, dry mouth, insomnia, dizziness, nausea
AE (sertraline): GI complaints, tremor, headache, insomnia, male sexual dysfunction
CI (SSRIs): Simultaneous treatment with MAO inhibitors, triptophan and oxitriptan; caution in children and adolescents < 18, hypersensitivity to product ingredients
CI (fluoxetine, in addition): Present or recent treatment with thioridazine
CI (fluvoxamine, in addit.): Coadministration of fexofenadine, astemizole or cisapride
CI (sertraline, in addition): Oral concentrate with disulfiram due to alcohol content

Citalopram	EHL 33–37h, Q0 >0.7, PRC C, Lact ?
Celexa *Tab 10mg, 20mg, 40mg Sol (oral) 10mg/5ml* **Generics** *Tab 10mg, 20mg, 40mg Sol (oral) 10mg/5ml*	**Depression:** Ini 20mg PO qd, incr to 40mg/d at an interval of >1wk, max 60mg/d DARF: To be used cautiously in renal impairment; see Prod Info

Escitalopram	EHL 27-32h, PRC C, Lact ?
Lexapro *Tab 5mg,10mg, 20mg, Sol (oral) 5mg/5ml*	**Depression:** 10mg PO qd, incr prn to 20mg/d DARF: To be used cautiously in severe renal impairment; see Prod Info

Fluoxetine	EHL 4-6d (chronic); 1-3d (acute), Q0 0.85, PRC C, Lact -
Prozac *Tab 10mg, Cap 10mg, 20mg, 40mg, Cap ext. rel 90mg, Sol (oral) 20mg/5ml* **Sarafem** *Cap 10mg, 20mg* **Generics** *Cap 10mg, 20mg, 40mg; Sol (oral) 20mg/5ml*	**Depression/obsessive compulsive DO:** Ini 20mg PO qam, incr prn q several wk, max 80mg/d; ext.rel.: 90mg PO once weekly; **bulimia:** 60mg PO qam DARF: See Prod Info

Fluvoxamine	EHL 15.6h, Q0 1.0, PRC C, Lact ?
Generics *Tab 25mg, 50mg, 100mg*	**Obsessive compulsive DO, depression:** Ini 50mg PO hs, incr prn by 50mg q4-7d (doses above 100mg/d: Div bid) max 300mg/d; **8-17y with obsessive compulsive DO:** Ini 25mg PO hs, incr prn by 25mg q4-7d (doses above 50mg/d: Div bid), max: 200mg/d; DARF: Low starting dosage + careful monitoring; see Prod Info

Paroxetine	EHL 17-22h, Q0 0.95, PRC C, Lact ?
Paxil *Tab 10mg, 20mg, 30mg, 40mg Susp 10mg/5ml* **Paxil CR** *Tab ext.rel. 12.5mg, 25mg, 37.5mg* **Generics** *Tab 10mg, 20mg, 30mg, 40mg*	**Depression:** Ini 20mg PO qam, incr prn by 10mg/d q 1wk, max 50mg/d; ext.rel.: Ini 25mg PO qam, incr prn by 12.5mg/d q 1wk, max 62.5mg/d; **obsessive compulsive DO:** Ini 20mg PO qam, incr by 10mg/d q 1wk, rec dosage 40mg/d, max 60mg/d; **panic DO:** Ini. 10mg/d qam; incr by 10mg/d, q 1wk, rec dosage 40mg/d, max 60mg/d; **social anxiety DO:** 20mg/d PO qam; DARF: Ini 10mg/d, max 40mg/d; for paroxetine ext. rel. ini 12.5mg/d, max 50mg/d

Sertraline	EHL 24h, Q0 1.0, PRC C, Lact ?
Zoloft *Tab 25mg, 50mg, 100mg, Conc (oral) 20mg/ml*	**Depression/obsessive compulsive DO:** Ini 50mg/d PO, prn gradually incr at 1wk intervals, max 200mg/d; **6-12 y/OCD:** 25mg/d PO, **13-17 y/OCD:** 50mg/d PO; **panic/post-traumatic stress DO:** Ini 25mg/d PO, incr after 1wk to 50mg/d, prn further incr q 1wk, max 200mg/d; **premenstrual dysphoric DO:** 50-100mg/d PO; DARF: Not req

12.1.8 Selective Serotonin Norepinephrine Reuptake Inhibitors (SSNRI)

MA: (duloxetine): Inhibition of serotonin and norepinephrine-reuptake ⇒ serotonin and norepinephrine levels in synaptic cleft ↑

AE (duloxetine): Fatigue, dizziness, headache, somnolence, tremor, insomnia, anxiety, suicidal ideation, worsening of depression, agitation, irritability, blurred vision, nausea, dry mouth, constipation, diarrhea, vomiting, decreased appetite, decreased libido, abnormal orgasm, erectile dysfunction, delayed ejaculation, dysuria, weight loss, increased sweating, rash, hot flushes

CI (duloxetine) hypersensitivity to d.; concomitant use of MAO inhibitors, uncontrolled narrow angle glaucoma

Duloxetine	EHL 12h, PRC C, Lact -
Cymbalta Cap ext.rel. 20mg, 30mg, 60mg	**Major depression DO:** 40-60mg/d PO qd or div bid; **diabetic peripheral neuropathic pain:** 60mg PO qd; **gen. anxiety DO:** Ini 30-60mg qd, may incr to max 120mg/d DARF: GFR (ml/min) <30: not rec DAHI: not rec

12.1.9 Serotonin Antagonists and Reuptake Inhibitors (SARI)

MA: Serotonin antagonists and reuptake inhib. (serotonin-5-HT$_2$ antagonists); trazodone: selective serotonin reuptake inhibitor, at low doses, trazodone appears to act as a serotonin antagonist and at higher doses as an agonist

AE (nefazodone): Dry mouth, nausea, somnolence, dizziness, blurred vision;

AE (trazodone): Dry mouth, dizziness, drowsiness, N/V, hypotension

CI (nefazodone): Hypersensitivity to phenylpiperazine antidepressants, administration of fexofenadine/astemizole/cisapride/MAOIs/pimozide/triazolam, caution with alprazolam, many other drug interactions

CI (trazodone): Hypersensitivity to trazodone, carcinoid syndrome, initial recovery phase of myocardial infarction

Nefazodone	EHL 1.9-5.3h, PRC C, Lact ?
Generics Tab 50mg, 100mg, 150mg, 200mg, 250mg	**Depression:** Ini 100mg PO bid, incr prn by 100-200mg/d, div bid, at >1wk intervals, maint 300-600mg/d div bid-tid

Trazodone	EHL 7.1h, Q0 1.0 (0.7), PRC C, Lact ?
Desyrel Tab 50mg, 100mg, 150mg, 300mg **Oleptro** Tab ext. rel. 150mg, 300mg **Generics** Tab 50mg, 100mg, 150mg, 300mg	**Depression:** 50-150mg/d PO in div doses, incr gradually prn by 50mg q3-4d, max 400mg/d div (outpatients), 600mg/d div (inpatients); ext.rel.: Ini 150mg PO qd, may incr by 75mg q3d, max 375mg/d; DARF: Not req

12.1.10 Norepinephrine Antagonist and Serotonin Antagonists (NASA)

MA: Norepinephrine antagonist and serotonin antagonist (norepinephrine, serotonin 5-HT$_2$ and 5-HT$_3$); **AE:** Drowsiness, dizziness, constipation, appetite↑, weight gain↑, dry mouth, agranulozytosis (0,1%); **CI:** Hypersensitivity to mirtazapine. Don't use with MAOIs

Mirtazapine — EHL 20-40h, PRC C, Lact ?

Remeron Tab 15mg, 30mg, 45mg **Remeron Soltab** Tab (orally disint) 15mg, 30mg, 45mg **Generics** Tab 7.5mg, 15mg, 30mg, 45mg; Tab (orally disint) 15mg, 30mg, 45mg	**Depression:** Ini 15mg/d PO, incr prn in intervals of >1-2wk to 15-45mg/d; DARF: See Prod Info

12.2 Antimanic (Bimodal) Drugs

MA/EF (lithium): Influence on phosphatidylinositol metabolism → Tx/PRO of manic depressive states, PRO of schizoaffective psychoses
MA (valproic acid): Inhibition of the enzymatic breakdown of GABA
MA (carbamazepine): Repeated stimulation of afferences ⇒ stimulus answer ↓
AE (lithium): Polydipsie, polyuria, GI disturbances, tremors, goiter, hypothyroidism, renal damage; **AE (valproic acid):** Tiredness, tremors, hair loss, hepatic damage, coagulation DO; **AE (carbamazepine):** Headache, dizziness, ataxia, dysopias, cholestatic hepatitis, disturbances of haematopoiesis, bradycardic cardiac arrhythmias, allergic reactions;
CI (lithium): Severe coronary dysfunction, M. Addison, RF
CI (valproic acid): Liver diseases in family, hypersensitivity to valproic acid; **CI (carbamazepine):** AV block, severe hepatic dysfunction, combination with MAO-inhib.

Lithium — EHL 14-24h, PRC D, Lact -, serum level(mEq/l):1-1.5 (acute), 0.6-1.2 (chronic)

Eskalith Cap 300mg; Tab ext.rel. 450mg **Lithobid** Tab ext.rel. 300mg **Generics** Cap 150mg, 300mg, Tab 300mg, Tab ext. rel 300mg, 450mg	**Acute mania:** 900-1800mg/d PO div bid-tid; **long-term use:** Maint 300mg PO tid-qid; ext.rel. 600mg bid; DARF: GFR (ml/min): > 50: 100%, 10-50: 50%-75%, < 10: 25%-50%

Valproic acid — EHL no data, PRC D, Lact + serum level: trough: 50-100µg/ml

Depacon Inj 100mg/ml **Depakene** Cap 250mg, Syr 250mg/5ml **Stavzor** Cap ext.rel. 125mg, 250mg, 500mg **Generics** Cap 250mg, Syr 250mg/5ml	**Mania:** Ini 750mg/d PO in divided doses, adjust dose rapidly to lowest therapeutic dose, max 60mg/kg/d; DARF: Not req.

Carbamazepine	EHL 12-17h (mult. dose), 25-65h (1x dose), Q0 1.0, PRC D, Lact +, serum-level (µg/ml): 4-12
Carbatrol Cap ext.rel. 100mg, 200mg, 300mg **Epitol** Tab (chew) 100mg, Tab 200mg **Equetro** Cap ext.rel. 100mg, 200mg, 300mg **Tegretol** Tab (chew) 100mg, Tab 200mg, Susp 100mg/5ml **Tegretol-XR** Tab (chew) 100mg, 200mg, 400mg **Teril** Tab 200mg; Sol (oral) 100mg/5ml **Generics** Tab (chew) 100mg, Tab 200mg; Tab 100mg, 200mg, 300mg, 400mg; Susp 100mg/5ml	**Mania:** 200mg PO qd-bid, incr by 200mg/d q2-4d, maint 600-1600mg/d, max 2,000-3,000mg/d; **epilepsy:** Ini 200mg PO bid, incr by 200mg/d qwk div tid-qid or bid (ext.rel.); maint 800-1,200mg/d, max 1,200mg/d, max 1,600mg/d; **CH** >12 y: Ini 200mg PO bid, or 100mg PO qid (susp), incr by 200mg/d qwk div tid-qid or bid (ext.rel.), max 1,000mg/d (age 12-15 y), max 1,200mg/d (age >15 y); **CH** 6-12 y: 100mg PO bid or 50mg PO qid (susp), incr by 100mg/d qwk div tid-qid or bid (ext.rel.), 15-30mg/kg/d PO div bid-qid, maint 400-800mg/d, max 1,000mg/d **CH** <6 y: 10-20mg/kg/d PO div bid-qid, max 35 mg/kg/d; **trigeminal neuralgia:** Ini 100mg PO bid or 200mg PO qd (ext. rel.) or 50mg PO qid (susp), incr by 200mg/d prn, maint 400-800mg/d, max 1,200mg/d; **migraine PRO:** 600mg/d, 10-20mg/kg/d PO div bid; DARF: Not req

12.3 Antipsychotics
12.3.1 Atypical - Serotonin Dopamine Receptor Antagonists (SDA)

AE (aripiprazole): Headache, anxiety, insomnia, lightheadedness, somnolence, akathisia, suicidal thoughts, seizures, bradycardia, nausea, vomiting, constipation, neuroleptic malignant syndrome, increased suicide risk; **AE** (clozapine): Agranulocytosis, sedation, salivation, CVS effects, dizziness/vertigo, seizures; **AE** (asenapine): Akathisia, oral hypoesthesia, and somnolence, dizziness, extrapyramidal symptoms other than akathisia, weight increased; **AE** (iloperidone): Dizziness, dry mouth, fatigue, nasal congestion, orthostatic hypotension, tachycardia, weight increased; **AE** (lurasidone): Somnolence, akathisia, nausea, parkinsonism, agitation; **AE** (olanzapine): somnolence, agitation, dizziness, constipation; **AE** (paliperidone): Headache, akathisia, somnolence, tachycardia, arrhythmia, QT-prolongation, neuroleptic malignant syndrome; **AE** (quetiapine): Somnolence, dizziness, dry mouth, constipation; **AE** (risperidone): Somnolence, dry mouth, constipation, blurred vision, extrapyramidal effects; **AE** (ziprasidone): Somnolence, akathisia, weight gain, dizziness, extrapyramidal symptoms; **CI** (aripiprazole): Hypersens. to arip.; **CI** (clozapine): Myeloproliferative DO, clozapine induced agranulocytosis uncontrolled epilepsy, coma, hypersensitivity to clozapine; **CI** (asenapine, iloperidone, olanzapine, quetiapine): Hypersensitivity to product ingredients; **CI** (lurasidone): Hypersens. to l., coadministration with strong CYP3A4 inhibitors (ketoconazole) or inducers (rifampin); **CI** (paliperidone): Hypersens. to p. or risperidone; **CI** (risperidone): Hyperprolactinemia, hypersens. to r.; **CI** (ziprasidone): QT-prolongat., hypersens. to z.

Aripiprazole	EHL 75-94h, PRC C, Lact -
Abilify *Tab* 2 mg, 5mg, 10mg, 15mg, 20mg, 30mg; *Tab (orally disint)* 10mg, 15mg, 20mg, 30mg; *Sol (oral)* 1mg/ml; *Inj* 9.75mg/1.3ml	**Schizophrenia:** Ini. 10-15mg PO qd, incr prn q2wk to max 30mg/d; **Bipolar DO:** Ini 30mg PO qd, maint 15-30mg; **Acute Agitation:** 9.75mg IM, may rep after 2h, max 30mg/d; DARF: not req

Asenapine	EHL 24h, PRC C, Lact ?
Saphris *Tab* 5mg, 10mg	**Schizophrenia:** Ini 5mg SL bid, maint. 5-10mg bid; **Bipolar DO:** Ini 10mg SL bid, maint. 5-10mg bid; **Bipolar DO adjunct to lithium or valproate:** Ini 5mg SL bid, maint 5-10mg bid; DARF: Not req

Clozapine	EHL 8-12h, Q0 1.0, PRC B, Lact -
Clozaril *Tab* 25mg, 100mg **Fazaclo** *Tab (orally disint)* 25mg, 50mg, 100mg **Generics** *Tab* 12.5mg, 25mg, 50mg, 100mg	**Tx-resistant schizophrenia:** Ini. 12.5mg PO qd-bid, incr by 25-50mg/d to 300-450mg/d (div bid-tid) by the end of 2wk, max 600-900mg/d

Iloperidone	EHL 18h, Q0 1.0, PRC C, Lact ?
Fanapt *Tab 1mg, 2mg, 4mg, 6mg, 8mg, 10mg, 12mg*	**Schizophrenia:** Ini 1mg PO bid x1d, then 2mg bid x1d, then incr. by 4 mg qd; max 24mg/d; DARF: Not req.; HD no data

Lurasidone	EHL 18h, Q0 >0.7, PRC B, Lact ?
Latuda *Tab 40mg, 80mg*	**Schizophrenia:** Ini 40mg PO qd, max 80mg/d; DARF: GFR (ml/min) 10-50: max 40mg/d

Olanzapine	EHL 21-54h (mean: 30h), Q0 >0.7, PRC C, Lact ?
Zyprexa *Tab 2.5mg, 5mg, 7.5mg, 10mg, 15mg; Inj 10mg/vial* **Zyprexa Zydis** *Tab (orally disint) 5mg, 10mg, 15mg, 20mg*	**Psychotic DO:** Ini 5-10mg PO qd, incr prn by 5mg/d qwk to usual effective dose of 10-15mg/d, max 20mg/d; **acute agitation:** 10mg IM, rep prn in 2 and 6h, 5mg in elderly, 2.5mg if debilitated; DARF: See Prod Info

Olanzapine + Fluoxetine	PRC C, Lact -
Symbyax *Cap 6 + 25mg, 6 + 50mg, 12 + 25mg, 12 + 50mg*	**Depressive episodes with bipolar DO:** Ini 6 + 25mg PO qd, incr prn to 12 + 50mg, max 18 + 75mg/d

Paliperidone	EHL 23h, PRC C, Lact -
Invega *Tab ext.rel. 3mg, 6mg, 9mg*	**Schizophrenia:** 6mg PO qam, incr prn 3mg/d q6d, max 12mg/d; DARF: GFR (ml/min) 50-79: max 6mg/d; 10-49: max 3mg/d

Quetiapine	EHL 6h, PRC C, Lact ?
Seroquel *Tab 25mg, 50mg, 100mg, 200mg, 300mg, 400mg*	**Psychotic DO:** Ini 25mg PO bid, incr by 25-50mg bid to 300-400mg/d (div bid-tid), range 150-750mg/d, max 800mg/d

Risperidone	EHL 20-30h, Q0 0.95 (0.1), PRC C, Lact ?
Risperdal *Tab 0.25mg, 0.5mg, 1mg, 2mg, 3mg, 4mg; Tab (orally disint) 0.5mg, 1mg, 2mg, 3mg, 4mg; Sol (oral) 1mg/ml* **Risperdal Consta** *Inj 25mg/vial, 37.5mg/vial, 50mg/vial*	**Schizoph:** Ini 1mg PO bid, incr prn by 1mg bid on d 2+d 3, then at intervals >1wk, maint 4-8mg/d, max 16mg/d; 25mg IM q2wk, incr prn to 37.5-50mg; **Bipolar Mania:** Ini 2-3mg PO, incr prn by 1mg/d, maint 1-6mg/d; DARF: Ini 0.5mg bid, incr prn by 0.5-1.5mg bid, then by 0.5mg bid qwk; see Prod Info; **Irritability with autistic DO:** CH >5Y; 15-20kg: d1-4 0.25mg PO d5-14 0.5mg, incr prn q2wk by 0.25mg/d, max 1mg; >20kg: d1-4 0.5mg PO d5-14 1mg, incr prn q2wk by 0.5mg/d, max 2.5mg if <45kg, max 3mg if > 45kg;

Ziprasidone	EHL 6-7h, PRC C, Lact -
Geodon *Tab* 20mg, 40mg, 60mg, 80mg *Susp (oral)* 10mg/ml, *Inj* 20mg/ml	**Schizoph.:** ini 20mg PO bid, incr prn q >2d to maint 20-80mg bid; **acute agitat.:** 10mg IM q2h prn, max 40mg/24h; DARF: not req

12.3.2 Antipsychotics: D_2 Antagonists – Low Potency

MA (D_2-Antagonists): Antagonism at central dopamine receptors; **EF** (D_2-Antagonists): Anti-psychotic and sedating (the higher the antipsychotic effect, the lower the sedating effect, and vice versa), sympatholytic, anticholinergic, antihista-minergic, antiserotoninergic; **AE** (D_2-Antagonists): Early and late dyskinesias, parkinsonism, acathisia, restlessness, excitement, depression, lethargy, hyperprolactinemia, amenorrhea, mydriasis, accommodation disturbances, difficult urination, constipation, glaucoma, rise in spasmophilia, HT, tachycardia, conduction disturbances, allergic reactions, complete blood count changes, cholestasis; **CI** (D_2-Antagonists): M. Parkinson, severe hepatic dysfunction, difficult urination, glaucoma, acute intoxications with sedating drugs; **AE** (chlorpromazine): HT, acathisia, tardive dyskinesia, arrhythmias, constipation; **AE** (mesoridazine): Tardive dyskinesia, drowsiness, seizures, dry mouth, myelosuppression; **AE** (thioridazine): Myelosuppression, arrhythmias, QT interval ↑, N/V, NMS, extrapyramidal effects; **CI** (chlorpromazine): Hypersens. to chlorpromazine, myelosuppression, coma; **CI** (thioridazine): Severe CNS depression, circulatory collapse, hypersens. to thioridazine products, HTN/HT/heart disease, QT interval ↑, patients on drugs that prolong the QT interval, patients on drugs that inhibit cytochrome p450-2D6; **CI** (mesoridazine): Hypersens. to mesoridazine products, coma

Chlorpromazine	EHL 6h, Q0 1.0, PRC C, Lact ?
Sonazine *Conc (oral)* 30mg/ml, 100mg/ml, *Syr* 10mg/5ml **Thorazine** *Cap ext.rel.* 200mg, 300mg, *Conc (oral)* 30mg/ml, 100mg/ml, *Syr* 10mg/5ml, *Supp* 25mg, 100mg, *Inj* 25mg/ml **Generics** *Tab* 10mg, 25mg, 50mg, 100mg, 200mg, *Conc (oral)* 30mg/ml, 100mg/ml, *Inj* 25mg/ml	**Psychotic DO:** Outpatients: Dose range 50-400mg/d; inpatients: Ini 25mg tid, incr gradually until effective dose is reached, max 800mg/d; **IM:** 25mg tid, can repeat with 25-50mg in 1h (severe cases: may be gradually incr over several d up to a max of 400mg q4-6h; a dose of 500mg/d is generally sufficient); **CH 6mo-12y: severe behavioral/psychotic DO:** 0.5mg/kg PO q4-6h prn or 1mg/kg PR q6-8h prn or 0.5mg/kg IM q6-8h prn

Thioridazine	EHL 21-24h , Q0 1.0, PRC C, Lact ?
Generics *Tab* 10mg, 15mg, 25mg, 50mg, 100mg, 150mg, 200mg, *Conc (oral)* 30mg/ml, 100mg/ml	**Psychotic DO:** Ini 50-100mg PO tid, gradual incr prn, maint 200-800mg/d div bid-qid, max 800mg/d; doses > 300mg/d are only rec for patients with severe psychoses **CH 2-12y (if unresponsive to other agents):** 0.5mg/kg/d PO div bid-tid, titrate to optimum clinical response or to max 3mg/kg/d

12.3.3 Antipsychotics: D$_2$ Antagonists - Mid Potency

MA, EF, AE, CI (D$_2$ Antagonists): See: Low potency neuroleptic drugs →208; **AE** (loxapine): Hypotension, extrapyramidal effects, blurred vision, weight ↑, sedation; **AE** (molindone): CVS effects, NMS, anticholinergic effects, extrapyramidal effect; **CI** (loxapine): coma, hypersensitivity to loxapine products; **CI** (molindone): Coma, hypersens. to m. products

Loxapine	EHL 4h (oral), 12h (IM), PRC C, Lact ?
Loxitane Cap 5mg, 10mg, 25mg, 50mg **Generics** Cap 5mg, 10mg, 25mg, 50mg	**Psychosis:** Ini 10mg PO bid or up to 50mg/d in severe cases, maint 60-100mg/d div bid-qid, max 250mg/d; IM: 12.5-50mg IM q4-12h, according to response

Molindone	EHL no data, PRC C, Lact ?
Moban Tab 5mg, 10mg, 25mg, 50mg	**Psychotic DO:** Ini 50-75mg/d PO, incr prn to 100mg/d after 3-4d, max 225mg/d; maint 5-15mg tid-qid (mild), 10-25mg tid-qid (moderate), up to 225mg/d (severe symptoms)

12.3.4 Antipsychotics: D$_2$ Antagonists - High Potency

MA, EF, AE, CI (D$_2$ Antagonists): See: Low potency neuroleptic drugs →208
AE (fluphenazine hydrochloride): Agranulocytosis, akathisia, weight gain, hepatotoxicity, extrapyramidal effects, neuroleptic malignant syndr.; **AE** (haloperidol): Sedation, dystonic/ extrapyramidal reactions, HT, arrhythmias; **AE** (perphenazine): Extrapyramidal, anticholinergic + CVS effects, seizures, sedation; **AE** (pimozide): Extrapyramidal + CVS effects, N, seizures; **AE** (thiothixene): Restlessness, blurred vision, extrapyramidal effects, N/V, myelosuppr.; **AE** (trifluoperazine): Seizures, NMS, extrapyramidal effects, blood dyscrasias; **CI** (fluphenazine): Coma, hypersensitivity to fluphenazine products; **CI** (haloperidol): Hypersensitivity to haloperidol products, Parkinson's disease; **CI** (perphenazine): Blood dyscrasias, subcortical brain damage, coma, hypersensitivity to perphenazine products, severe liver disease; **CI** (pimozide): QT interval ↑, concomitant macrolides, hypersensitivity to pimozide, coma; **CI** (thiothixene): Hypersensitivity to thiothixene products; **CI** (trifluoperazine): Coma, bone marrow depression, hypersensitivity to trifluoperazine

Fluphenazine hydrochloride	EHL 33h, PRC C, Lact ?
Prolixin Tab 1mg, 2.5mg, 5mg, 10mg, Conc (oral) 5mg/ml, Elixir 2.5mg/5ml, Inj 2.5mg/ml **Generics** Tab 1mg, 2.5mg, 5mg, 10mg, Conc (oral) 5mg/ml, Elixir 2.5mg/5ml, Inj 2.5mg/ml	**Psychosis:** 0.5-10mg/d PO div q6-8h; usual effective doses 1-20mg/d, max 40mg/d PO; **IM:** 1.25-10mg/d div q6-8h, max 10mg/d

Haloperidol	EHL 21h, IM: approx. 3wk, Q0 1.0, PRC C, Lact ?
Haldol *Inj 5mg/ml (Lactat), 50mg/ml (Decanoat), 100mg/ml (Decanoat)* **Generics** *Tab 0.5mg, 1mg, 2mg, 5mg, 10mg; Conc (oral) 2mg/ml; Sol (oral) 1mg/ml; Inj 5mg/ml (Lactat), 50mg/ml (Decanoat), 100mg/ml (Decanoat)*	**Acutely agitated patients:** Ini 2-5mg IM, may repeat q1-8h; **psychotic DO:** Ini 1-6mg/d PO (moderate) and 6-15mg/d (severe symptoms) div bid-tid; usual range 1-15mg/d, max100mg/d; **Haldol decanoate** (oral to depot conversion): Ini: 10-20 x the previous daily oral dose IM, but 100mg max ini dose, at monthly intervals; **CH 3-12 y psychotic DO:** 0.05-0.15mg/kg/d PO div bid-tid, **non-psychotic DO:** 0.05-0.075mg/kg/d PO div bid-tid; **DARF:** Not req
Perphenazine	EHL 8.4-12.3h, Q0 1.0, PRC C, Lact -
Generics *Tab 2mg, 4mg, 8mg, 16mg; Conc (oral) 16mg/5ml*	**Psychotic symptoms:** Ini 4-8mg PO tid (moderately disturbed outpatients) or 8-16mg PO bid-qid (inpatients); IM: Ini 5-10mg IM, then 5mg IM q6h prn, max 15mg/d IM (out-), max 30mg/d IM (inpatients)
Pimozide	EHL 53-55h, Q0 1.0, PRC C, Lact ?
Orap *Tab 1mg, 2mg*	**Tourette's syndrome:** Ini 1-2mg/d PO in div doses, incr q2d prn; max 0.2mg/kg/d up to 10mg/d; **CH >12y:** Ini 0.05mg/kg PO hs, incr prn q3d to max 0.2mg/kg up to 10mg/d; DARF: probably not req; see Prod Info
Thiothixene	EHL 34h, PRC C, Lact ?
Navane *Cap 1mg, 2mg, 5mg, 10mg, 20mg, Conc (oral) 5mg/ml, Inj 10mg/vial* **Generics** *Cap 1mg, 2mg, 5mg, 10mg, Conc (oral) 5mg/ml*	**Schizophrenia:** Ini 6mg PO div tid (milder conditions) and 5mg bid (severe conditions); usual effective dose range 20-30mg/d, max 60mg/d; IM: Ini 4mg bid-qid, max 30mg/d
Trifluoperazine	EHL 24h, PRC C, Lact ?
Stelazine *Tab 1mg, 2mg, 5mg, 10mg, Conc (oral) 10mg/ml, Inj 2mg/ml* **Generics** *Tab 1mg, 2mg, 5mg, 10mg*	**Non-psychotic anxiety:** 1-2mg PO bid for up to 12wk, max 6mg/d; **psychotic DO:** Ini 2-5mg PO bid, usual dose is 15-20mg/d, sometimes up to 40mg/d; IM: 1-2mg q4-6h prn; **CH 6-12y** (hospitalized or under close supervision): 1mg PO qd-bid, prn gradually incr, max 15mg/d; IM: 1mg IM qd-bid

12.4 Anxiolytics, Hypnotics
12.4.1 Benzodiazepines

MA: Opening of Cl⁻ channels ⇒ inhibition of GABA neurons↑, especially in limbic system
EF: Sedative, sleep inducing, anxiolytic, anti-aggressive, anti-convulsive, muscle relaxing
AE: Tiredness, sleepiness, drowsiness, confusion, paradox reactions, anterograde amnesia, respiratory depression, psychic and physical addiction
CI: Myasthenia gravis, severe hepatic damage, respiratory insufficiency, ataxia

Alprazolam	EHL 11.23h, Q0 >0.7, PRC D, Lact ?
Niravam Tab (orally disint) 0.25mg, 0.5mg, 1mg, 2mg **Xanax** Tab 0.25mg, 0.5mg, 1mg, 2mg ; Tab ext. rel 0.5mg, 1mg, 2mg, 3mg **Generics** Tab 0.25mg, 0.5mg, 1mg, 2mg, Conc (oral) 1mg/ml	**Anxiety** Ini 0.25-0.5mg PO tid, incr prn q3-4d to max 4mg/d, usual effective dose 0.5-4mg/d in div dose **panic DO:** Ini 0.5mg PO tid, incr prn by max 1mg/d q3-4d, slower titration may be needed at doses > 4mg/d, usual effective dose 1-10mg/d (mean 5-6mg/d), max 10mg/d

Chlordiazepoxide	EHL 10-48h, Q0 1.0 (1.0), PRC D, Lact ?
Librium Cap 5mg, 10mg, 25mg **Generics** Cap 5mg, 10mg, 25mg	**Anxiety:** Usual oral dose range is 5-10mg PO tid-qid (mild to moderate anxiety + tension) or 20-25mg tid-qid (severe anxiety + tension); **IV/IM: Acute or severe anxiety:** 25-50mg IM/IV tid-qid; **CH > 6y + anxiety:** Ini with lowest dose, incr prn, maint 5mg PO bid-qid, max 10mg bid-tid; **acute alcohol withdrawal:** 50-100mg IM/IV, repeat q2-4h prn up to 300mg/d DARF: mild to moderate RF: Not req; CrCl (ml/min) <10: 50%; see Prod Info

Clonazepam	EHL 30-40h, PRC C, Lact-serum-level (ng/ml): 25-30
Klonopin Tab 0.125mg, 0.25mg, 0.5mg, 1mg, 2mg, Tab (orally disint) 0.125mg, 0.25mg, 0.5mg, 1mg, 2mg **Generics** Tab 0.5mg, 1mg, 2mg; Tab (orally disint) 0.125mg, 0.25mg, 0.5mg, 1mg, 2mg	**Panic DO:** Ini 0.25mg PO bid, gradually incr prn after 3d, max 4mg/d; (gradually decr by 0.125mg twice daily, q3d);

Clorazepate	EHL 2.29h, PRC D, Lact ?
Gen-xene Tab 3.75mg, 7.5mg, 15mg **Tranxene** Tab 3.75mg, 7.5mg, 15mg **Tranxene sd** Tab 11.25mg, 22.5mg **Generics** Cap 3.75mg, 7.5mg, 15mg	**Anxiety:** ini 7.5-15mg PO, maint. 15-60mg/d according to patients response; DARF: Not req

Diazepam	EHL 0.83-2.25d, Q0 1.0 (1.0), PRC D, Lact ?
Diastat Gel (rectal) 2.5mg/0.5ml, 10mg/2ml, 20mg/4ml **Diazepam Intensol** Conc (oral) 5mg/ml **Valium** Tab 2mg, 5mg, 10mg; **Generics** Tab 2mg, 5mg, 10mg, Sol (oral) 5mg/5ml / Inj 5mg/ml	**Anxiety:** 2-10mg PO bid-qid; IM/IV: 2-5mg IM/IV, repeat in 3-4h prn (moderate anxiety); 5-10mg IM/IV, repeat q3-4h prn (severe DO); DARF: See Prod Info; **epilepsy: muscle spasm:** 2-10mg bid-qid

Estazolam	EHL 10-24h, PRC X, Lact ?
Prosom Tab 1mg, 2mg **Generics** Tab 1mg, 2mg	**Insomnia:** 1-2mg PO hs prn, reduce dose to 0.5mg in elderly, small, debilitated patients, incr prn with caution; DARF: Not req

Flurazepam	EHL 2.3h, Q0 1.0 (0.7), PRC X, Lact ?
Dalmane Cap 15mg, 30mg **Generics** Cap 15mg, 30mg	**Short term Tx of insomnia:** 15-30mg PO hs; DARF: See Prod Info

Lorazepam	EHL 10-20h (mean 12h) , Q0 1.0, PRC D, Lact ?
Ativan Tab 0.5mg, 1mg, 2mg; Inj 2mg/ml, 4mg/ml **Generics** Tab 0.5mg, 1mg, 2mg, Sol (oral) 0.5mg/5ml, Conc (oral) 2mg/ml, Inj 2mg/ml, 4mg/ml	**Anxiety:** Ini 0.5-1mg PO/IM/IV bid-tid, maint 2-6mg/d in div doses, max 10mg/d (div) **insomnia:** 2-4mg PO hs prn **N/V with Chemo:** 2.5mg PO/IM/IV DARF: Avoid use

Oxazepam	EHL 2.8-8.6h, Q0 1.0, PRC D, Lact ?
Generics Cap 10mg, 15mg, 30mg	**Anxiety:** 10-15mg PO tid-qid (mild-to-moderate anxiety), 15-30mg tid-qid (severe anxiety and agitation with depression); **alcohol withdrawal:** 15-30mg tid-qid; DARF: Not req, see Prod Info

Temazepam	EHL 3.5-18.4h, Q0 1.0, PRC X, Lact ?
Restoril Cap 7.5mg, 15mg, 22.5mg, 30mg **Generics** Cap 15mg, 30mg	**Insomnia:** 7.5-30mg PO hs

Triazolam	EHL 2.3h, Q0 1.0, PRC X, Lact ?
Halcion Tab 0.125mg, 0.25mg **Generics** Tab 0.125mg, 0.25mg	**Insomnia:** 0.125-0.25mg PO hs prn, max 0.5mg/d

12.4.2 Sedating Antihistamines

MA (diphenhydramine): Antihistamine with sedative and hypnotic effect (see other antihistamines)
AE (diphenhydramine): Dizziness, headache, convulsions, cardiac arrhythmia, oral dryness, micturition disturbances, paralytic ileus
CI (diphenhydramine): Glaucoma, prostate hypertrophy with residual urine, acute asthma attacks, pheochromocytoma, epilepsy

Diphenhydramine	EHL 4-8h (prolonged with age), Q0 0.9, PRC B, Lact -
Benadryl Inj 50mg/ml Generics Cap 25mg, 50mg, Elixir 12.5mg/5ml, Inj 10mg/ml, 50mg/ml	Insomnia: 50mg PO hs; DARF: GFR (ml/min) >50: q6h, 10-50: q6-12h, < 10: q12-18h; see Prod Info

12.4.3 Barbiturates

MA (barbiturat.): Reinforcement of the inhibitory effect caused by GABA in the CNS
EF (barbiturates): Sedative, sleep inducing, anxiolytic, anti-aggressive, anti-convulsive, muscle relaxing; **AE** (barbiturates): Tiredness, dizziness, anterograde amnesia, ataxia, dysopias, porphyria, N/V, hepatic dysfunction, bradycardia, respiratory depression, skin reactions, complete blood count changes, enzyme induction, addiction; **AE** (butabarbital): Somnolence, agitation, confusion, dizziness, hypoventilation; **AE** (pentobarbital): Respiratory depression, tachycardia, myasthenia gravis, drowsiness; **AE** (secobarbital): Vertigo, excitation, respiratory depression, CNS depression; **CI** (barbiturates): Porphyria, severe hepatic/renal dysfunction, status asthmaticus, respirat. insufficiency, barbiturate sensitivity

Butabarbital	EHL 34-100h, PRC D, Lact ?
Butisol Sodium Tab 30mg, 50mg, Elixir (oral) 30mg/5ml Generics Tab 16.2mg, 30mg, 32.4mg	Sedation: 15-30mg PO tid-qid insomnia: 50-100mg PO hs prn

Pentobarbital	EHL 15-48h, PRC D, Lact ?
Nembutal Sodium Inj 50mg/ml	Barbiturate coma: Ini 10-15mg/kg IV over 1-2h, then 1mg/kg/h

Secobarbital	EHL 19-34h, PRC D, Lact +
Seconal Sodium Cap 50mg, 100mg Generics Cap 100mg	Insomnia: 100mg PO hs prn; DARF: Not req

12.4.4 Other Anxiolytics, Hypnotics

MA (buspirone): Unknown, high affinity for 5-HT$_{1A}$-receptors; **MA** (eszopiclone): Interaction with GABA-receptor complexes; **MA** (ramelteon): Binds to melatonin 1 and 2-receptors ⇒ sleep induction; **MA** (zaleplon, zolpidem): benzodiazepine-like effect; **AE** (buspirone): Sedation, dizziness; **AE** (eszopiclone): Dizziness, headache, somnolence, unpleasant taste, respiratory infection; **AE** (ramelteon): Dizziness, somnolence, depression, worsened insomnia, headache, fatigue, nausea, diarrhea, impaired taste, arthralgia, myalgia, upper respiratory tract infx, influenza, decreased cortisol levels, decreased testosterone levels , increased prolactin levels, galactorrhea, amenorrhea; **AE** (zaleplon, zolpidem): allergic reactions, tiredness, headache, dizziness, somnolence, nausea, development of addiction; **CI** (buspirone): Hypersens. to buspirone products; **CI** (eszopiclone): None known; **CI** (ramelteon): Hypersens. to r.; severe hepatic impairment, combination w/fluvoxamine; **CI** (zaleplon, zolpidem): Myasthenia gravis, severe liver impairment, hypersens. to product ingredients

Buspirone	EHL 2.4-2.7h, Q0 1.0, PRC B, Lact ?
Buspar *Tab 5mg, 10mg, 15mg, 30mg* **Generics** *Tab 5mg, 7.5mg, 10mg, 15mg*	**Anxiety:** Ini 7.5mg PO bid, incr by 5mg/d q2-3d prn, usual effective dose 20-30mg/d (in div doses), max 60mg/d DARF: See Prod Info

Eszopiclone	EHL 6h, PRC C, Lact ?
Lunesta *Tab 1mg, 2mg, 3mg*	**Insomnia:** Ini 2mg PO hs, incr prn to 3mg; elderly: 1-2mg; DARF: Not req

Ramelteon	EHL 1-2.6h, PRC C, Lact ?
Rozerem *Tab 8mg*	**Insomnia:** 8mg PO hs ; DARF: Not req

Zaleplon	EHL 1h, Q0 1.0, PRC C, Lact -
Sonata *Cap 5mg, 10mg*	**Short-term Tx of insomnia:** 5-10mg PO hs prn; DARF: See Prescr.Info

Zolpidem	EHL 2-2.6h, Q0 1.0, PRC B, Lact ?
Ambien *Tab 5mg, 10mg* *Tab ext. rel. 6.25mg, 12.5mg* **Tovalt** *Tab (orally disint) 5mg, 10mg* **Generics** *Tab 5mg, 10mg*	**Insomnia:** 5-12.5mg PO hs prn (limit to 7-10d), max 12.5mg PO; DARF: Not req

12.4.5 Anxiolytics, Hypnotics - Combinations

AE (amitriptyline + chlordiazepoxide): Drowsiness, anticholinergic + CVS effects, seizures, myelosuppression
AE (perphenazine): Extrapyramidal, anticholinergic + CVS effects, sedation, seizures;
CI (amitriptyline + chlordiazepoxide): Hypersens. to benzodiazepines or TCAs, concomitant use with MAO inhib., recovery following an MI
CI (amitriptyline + perphenazine): CVS disease, recovery period after MI, MAO Inhib. usage, large doses of other CNS depressants, blood dyscrasias, bone marrow depression/hepatic damage, hypersens. to perphenazine, other piperazine phenothiazines, amitriptyline, or other TCA, subcortical brain damage, coma

Chlordiazepoxide + Amitriptyline	
Limbitrol, Generics *Tab 5mg + 12.5mg, 10mg + 25mg,*	**Anxiety/depression:** 1 Tab PO tid-qid, max 6 Tab/d; DARF see Prod Info

Perphenazine + Amitriptyline	
Generics *Tab 2mg + 10mg, 4mg + 10mg, 2mg + 25mg, 4mg + 25mg, 4mg + 50mg*	**Depression/anxiety:** Ini 2-4mg perphen. + 25mg amitript. tid-qid, use lowest effective level for maint; max daily dose 16mg perphenazine + 200mg amitriptyline

12.5 Drugs Used in Substance Dependence
12.5.1 Smoking Cessation

MA/EF (bupropion): Catecholamine reuptake in CNS ↓ ⇒ local concentrations of noradrenaline + dopamine ↑ ⇒ nicotine withdrawal symptoms ↓, urge to smoke ↓
MA/EF (nicotine products): Ganglionic (nicotinic) cholinergic-receptor agonists; used for nicotine replacement therapy as temporary adjunct in cessation of cigarette smoking;
MA (varenicline): Binds to nicotine receptors
AE (nicotine prod.): Tachycardia, diarrhea, nausea/indigestion, dizziness, insomnia, headache, nasal irritation with spray, skin irritation with patch, mouth irritation (gum)
AE (bupropion): Fever, oral dryness, N/V, stomachache, constipation, insomnia, difficulty concentrating, headache, tachycardia, BP ↑, depression, restlessness, fear, seizures/tremors, agitation, insomnia, hypersens. reactions; **AE (varenicline):** Headache, insomnia, abnormal dreams, somnolence, lethargy, fatigue, malaise, asthenia, altered taste, N/V, abdominal pain, flatulence, dyspepsia, constipation, dry mouth, increased appetite, anorexia, dyspnea, upper respiratory infxns, rash;
CI (nicotine products): Angina, arrhythmias, active temporomandibular joint disease (gum), immediately post-MI, continued use of tobacco prod., gastric ulcer, uncontrolled HTN, hypersens. to nicotine prod.; **CI (bupropion):** Epilepsy, bulimia, anorexia, bipolar psychosis, severe liver cirrhosis, comb. with MAO inhib., children/adolescents < 18, hypersens. to bupropion prod., concomitant use of other bupropion products
CI (varenicline): Hypersensitivity to v.

Bupropion	EHL 14h (chronic dosing 21h), Q0 >0.8, PRC B, Lact ?	
Zyban *Tab ext.rel. 150mg*		**Smoking cessation:** Ini 150mg PO qd x 3d, incr to 150mg PO bid x 7-12wk, max 150mg PO bid; **depression →200** ; **DARF:** See Prod Info
Nicotine gum	EHL 30-120min, PRC C, Lact ?	
Nicorette *Gum (chew, buccal) 2mg, 4mg*		**Smoking cessation:** 1 piece (2mg) q1-2h for 6wk, then 1 piece (2mg) q2-4h for 3wk, then 1 piece (2mg) q4-8h for 3wk, max 30 pieces/d of 2mg or 24 pieces/d of 4mg; 4mg pieces for high cigarette use (> 24 cigarettes/d)
Nicotine inhalation system	PRC D, Lact ?	
Nicotrol *Inhalant 4mg/cartridge*		**Smoking cessation:** 6-16 cartridges/d x 12wk, then reduction; max. 16 cartridges/d
Nicotine nasal spray	PRC D, Lact ?	
Nicotrol *Spray (nasal) 0.5mg/Spray*		**Smoking cessation:** 1-2 doses/h (each dose = 2 sprays, 1 in each nostril), max 5doses/h or 40 doses/24h

Nicotine patches	PRC D, Lact ?
Habitrol Film (ext.rel, TD) 7mg/24h, 14mg/24h, 21mg/24h **Nicoderm** Film (ext.rel, TD) 7mg/24h, 14mg/24h, 21mg/24hr **Generics** Film (ext.rel, TD) 7mg/24h, 14mg/24h, 21mg/24h	**Smoking cessation:** See Prod Info

Varenicline	EHL 24h, PRC C, Lact ?
Chantix Tab 0.5mg, 1mg	**Smoking cessation:** 0.5mg PO qd d1-3, 0.5mg bid d4-7, then 1mg bid d8-wk12, stop smoking d8, max 2mg/d; DARF: GFR (ml/min) <30: max 0.5mg bid; HD: 0.5mg qd

12.5.2 Alcohol Dependence

MA/EF (acamprosate): Unknown, interaction with glutamate and GABA neurotransmitters
MA/EF (disulfiram): Enzymatic oxid. of acetaldehyde to acetate ↓, during normal alcohol catabolism ⇒ acetaldehyde ↑ ⇒ unpleasant sympt., hypersens. to alc.
AE (acamprosate): Suicidality, depression, diarrhea, insomnia, anxiety, asthenia, nausea, pruritus, dizziness, tremor, abdom. pain, back pain, chest pain, flu syndr., chills
AE (disulfiram): Psychotic reactions, neuropathy, blurred vision, seizures, hepatitis
CI (acamprosate): Hypersens. to a., GFR < 30 ml/min; **CI** (disulfiram): Hypersensitivity to disulfiram, recent use of paraldehyde, metronidazole, ethanol, exposure to ethylene dibromide (pesticides), myocard. disease, psychoses

Acamprosate	EHL 20-33h PRC C, Lact ?
Campral Tab 333mg	**Maintenance of abstinence from alcohol:** 666mg tid PO; DARF (ml/min): 30-50: 333mg tid; <30: contraind.

Disulfiram	EHL 12h, Q0 0.5, PRC C, Lact ?
Antabuse Tab 250mg	**Alcoholism:** Ini up to max 500mg/d PO for 1-2wk, maint 125-250mg/d, max 500mg/d

see Diazepam→211, Chloral Hydrate→213, Chlordiazepoxide→211, Oxazepam→211

12.5.3 Opioid Dependence

AE (methadone): Respiratory depression, dizziness, N/V, sweating, constipation
AE (naltrexone): Opioid withdrawal-like syndr., nausea, headache, dizziness, anxiety
CI (methadone): Hypersensitivity to methadone; **CI** (naltrexone): Concomitant opioid analgesics, opioid dependency or withdrawal, hypersensitivity to naltrexone, acute hepatitis or liver failure

Methadone	EHL 23h (IV), 22h (chronic PO), PRC C, Lact ?
Dolophine HCT *Tab 5mg, 10mg, Syr (oral) 10mg/30ml* **Methadose** *Tab 5mg, 10mg, Tab (dispersible) 40mg, Conc (oral) 10mg/ml* **Generics** *Tab 5mg, 10mg, Tab (dispersible) 40mg, Conc (oral) 10mg/ml, Sol (oral) 5mg/5ml, 10mg/5ml*	**Narcotic addiction:** 40-180mg/d PO (div), taper dose as appropriate to avoid withdrawal symptoms DARF: See Prod Info, (GFR (ml/min): > 50: q6h; 10-50: q8h, severe RF: q8-12h)

Naltrexone	EHL 4h (PO), 5-10d (IM), Q0 1.0, PRC C, Lact ?
Revia *Tab 50mg* **Vivitrol** *Inj 380mg/vial* **Generics** *Tab 25mg, 50mg, 100mg*	**Alcohol dependence:** 50mg PO qd or 380mg IM q4wk; **narcotic dependence:** Ini 25mg PO qd, incr to 50mg PO qd if no signs of withdrawal

12.6 CNS Stimulants

MA/EF (amphetamine): CNS/respiratory stimulation; sympathomimetic activity ↑ ⇒ pressor response, mydriasis, bronchodilation, contraction of urinary bladder sphincter; **MA/EF** (armodafinil): Unknown; wake-promoting actions similiar to symathomimetics; **MA/EF** (atomoxetine): Selective inhibition of norepinephrine reuptake; **MA/EF** (caffeine): competitive inhibition of phosphodiesterase ⇒ intracellular cyclic AMP ↑ ⇒ CNS stimulation at all levels (thought flow ↑, wakefulness); **MA/EF** (clonidine): Stimulates alpha-2-receptors, exact MA unknown; **MA/EF** (methylphenidate): Amphetamine derivate → release of catecholamines ⇒ centrally stimulating; **MA/EF** (modafinil): Potentiation of cerebral α_1-adrenergic activity ⇒ improvement of vigilance ↑, number of sudden sleep episodes ↓ **MA/EF** (Pemoline): CNS and respiratory stimulation and weak sympathomimetic activity;

AE (amphetamine): Restlessness, palpitations/tachycardia, dizziness, HTN; **AE** (armodafinil): Headache, N/V, dizziness, insomnia, diarrhea, depression, anxiety, dry mouth, fatigue, Stevens-Johnson-Syndrome, flulike syndrome; **AE** (atomoxetine): Headache, insomnia, dry mouth, nausea, decreased appetite, constipation, upper abdominal pain, vomiting, cough **AE** (caffeine): Restlessness, vomiting, tachycardia; **AE** (clonidine): Somnolence, fatigue, URTI, throat pain, insomnia, nightmares, emotional DO, constipation, nasal congestion, dry mouth, ear pain, increased body temperature; **AE** (dextroamphetamine): Insomnia, tachycardia, dry mouth, dependence, anorexia; **AE** (lisdexamfetamine): Insomnia, irritability, headache, fever, tics, psychomotor hyperactivity, initial insomnia, dizziness, somnolence, affect lability, ventricular hypertrophy, N/V, abdominal pain, decreased appetite, dry mouth, decreased weight, rash; **AE** (methylphenidate): Restlessness, behavior DO, slurred speech, dermatitis, skin rashes, convulsions, insomnia, states of excitability, psychoses, development of addiction; **AE** (modafinil): Headache, nausea, nervousness, loss of appetite, sleep DO; **AE** (pemoline): Anorexia, insomnia, dizziness, LFT abnormalities, Tourette's syndrom; **AE** (sodium oxybate): Headche, nausea, dizziness, pain, somnolence, pharyngitis, infection, flu-syndrome; **CI** (amphetamine): MAOI therapy, drug abuse, HTN, glaucoma, CAD, hyperthyroidism

CI (armodafinil): Hypersens. to a. ; **CI** (atomoxetine): Hypersens. to atom., MAOI therapy, narrow angle glaHucoma; **CI (clonidine): hypersens. to c.;** **CI** (dextroamphetamine): ypersens. to d., concomitant MAOI, CVS disease, hyperthyroidism; **CI** (lisdexamfetamine): Hypersens. to l., patients with history of drug abuse or agitated states and within 14d of using an MAO inhibitor; **CI** (methylphenidate): Glaucoma, marked anxiety, tension, agitation, depression, psychoses, addictions, hypersens. to methylphenidate, hyperthyroidism, prostate hypertrophy, pheochromocytoma; **CI** (modafinil): Combination with prazosin, addictions; **CI** (pemoline): Hypersens. to pemoline, liver disease, ADD with concomitant Tourette's syndrome/tics; **CI** (sodium oxybate): Treatment with sedative hypnotic agents, succinic semialdehyde dehydrogenase deficiency

Amphetamine + Dextroamphetamine	
Adderall *Tab 2.5 + 2.5mg, 3.75 + 3.75mg, 6.25 + 6.25mg, 10 + 10mg, 15 + 15mg; Tab ext.rel. 5 + 5mg, 10 + 10mg, 15 + 15mg*	**Narcolepsy:** 5-60mg/d in div doses, **CH 6-12y:** Ini 5mg PO qd, incr by 5mg qwk prn; **>12y:** Ini 10mg PO qd, incr by 10mg qwk prn; **attention deficit DO, hyperactivity: CH 3-5y:** Ini 2.5mg PO qd, incr by 2.5mg qwk prn; **age >6y:** Ini 5mg PO qd-bid, incr by 5mg qwk prn; max 40mg/d; ext.rel.: Ini 10mg PO qd, incr prn by 10mg qwk, max 30mg/d; DARF: See Prod Info
Armodafinil	EHL 15h, PRC C, Lact ?
Nuvigil *Tab 50mg, 150mg, 250mg*	**Sleepiness with OSAHS, narcolepsy:** 150-250mg PO qd; shift work sleep disorder: 150mg qd;
Atomoxetine	EHL 22h, PRC C, Lact ?
Strattera *Cap 10mg, 18mg, 25mg, 40mg, 60mg, 80mg, 100mg*	**Attention deficit hyperactivity DO:** >70kg: Ini 40mg/d PO, incr after 3d to 80mg/d div qd-bid; max 100mg/d after 2-4wk; <70kg: Ini 0.5mg/kg/d PO, incr. after 3d to 1.2mg/kg/d div qd-bid; max 1.4mg/d DARF: not req
Caffeine	EHL 4-5h, PRC C, Lact +
Caffedrine *Cap ext. rel. 200mg* **NoDoz** *Tab 100mg, 200mg, Tab (chew) 100mg* **Vivarin** *Tab 200mg*	**Fatigue:** 100-200mg PO q3-4h prn
Clonidine	EHL 12-16h, PRC C, Lact +
Kapvay *Tab ext.rel. 0.1mg, 0.2mg*	**Attention deficit hyperactivity DO:** Ini 0.1mg PO qd, incr prn by 0.1mg/d qwk; divide dose bid, max 0.4mg/d
Dextroamphetamine	EHL 7-34h, PRC C, Lact -
Dexedrine *Tab 5mg, Cap ext.rel. 5mg, 15mg, 10mg* **Dextrostat** *Tab 5mg, 10mg* **Generics** *Tab 5mg, 10mg*	**Narcolepsy:** Usual 5-60mg/d (div. qd-tid) **6-12y + narcolepsy:**lini 5mg/d PO, incr qwk by 5mg prn; **>12y:** Ini 10mg PO qd, incr qwk by 10mg/d prn; **attention deficit hyperactivity DO:** 3-5y: Ini 2.5mg PO qd, incr by 2.5mg qwk prn; **6y:** Ini 5mg PO qd-bid, incr by 5mg qwk prn, max 40mg/d div qd-tid at 4-6h intervals

Dexmethylphenidate	EHL 2.2h, PRC C, Lact ?
Focalin *Tab 2.5mg, 5mg, 10mg, Cap (ext.rel.) 5mg, 10mg, 20mg*	**Attention deficit hyperactivity DO:** 6-17y: Ini 2.5mg PO bid, incr by 2.5-5mg qwk prn to max 10mg bid

Lisdexamfetamine	EHL 10.1h
Vyvanse *Cap 30mg, 50mg, 70mg*	**Attention deficit hyperactivity DO:** 6-12y: Ini 30mg PO qd, incr prn by 20mg qwk prn to max 70mg/d;

Methylphenidate	EHL PO 2-7h; IV 1-2h, Q0 0.95, PRC C, Lact ?
Concerta *Tab (ext.rel.) 18mg, 27mg, 36mg, 54mg* **Daytrana** *Film (ext.rel ,TD) 10mg/9h, 15mg/9h, 20mg/9h, 30mg/9h* **Metadate ER** *Tab (ext.rel.) 10mg, 20mg* **Metadate CD** *Cap (ext.rel.)10mg, 20mg, 30mg, 40mg, 50mg, 60mg* **Methylin** *Tab (chew) 2.5mg, 5mg, 10mg; Sol (oral) 5mg/5ml, 10mg/5ml* **Methylin ER** *Tab (ext.rel.) 10mg, 20mg* **Ritalin** *Tab 5mg, 10mg, 20mg; Tab ext.rel 10mg, 20mg, 30mg, 40mg* **Generics** *Tab 5mg, 10mg, 20mg*	**Narcolepsy:** Narcolepsy 10-60mg/d in 2-3 div doses (mean 20-30mg/d); **attention deficit DO: CH > 6y:** Ini 2.5-5mg PO bid before breakfast and lunch, incr gradually by 5-10mg qwk prn to max 60mg/d; apply one patch 2h before desired effect and remove 9h later, incr dose qwk prn, max 30mg/d;

Modafinil	EHL 7.5-15h, PRC C, Lact ?
Provigil *Tab 100mg, 200mg*	**Narcolepsy:** 200mg PO qam; DARF: Ini 100-200mg/d, gradual incr based on safety and tolerability, see Prod Info

Sodium oxybate	EHL 22min, PRC B, Lact ?
Xyrem *Sol (oral) 500mg/ml*	**Cataplexy with narcolepsy:** To be taken at bedtime and 2.5-4h later, ini 4.5g/d, may incr. to max. 9g/d in increments of 1.5g/d; DARF not req

13 Appendix

13.1 List of Abbreviations

≥	greater than or equal to
<	less than
>	greater than
+/-	plus or minus
%	percent
5 HT	5-hydroxytryptamine (Serotonin)
AAPs	atypical antipsychotics
AAS	anabolic androgenic steroids
ABG	arterial blood gas
AD	antidepressants
ADHD	attention deficit hyperactivity disorder
AIMS	abnormal involuntary movement scale
AN	anorexia nervosa
AP	antipsychotics
ARP	aripiprazole
ASD	acute stress disorder
ASDS	acute stress disorder scale
AUDIT	alcohol use disorders identification test
B12	cobalamin
BARS	barnes-akathisia rating scale
BED	binge eating disorder
BLIPS	brief limited intermittent psychotic symptoms
BMI	body mass index
BN	bulimia nervosa

BPD	borderline personality disorder
BUN	blood urea nitrogen
Ca	calcium
CAARMS	comprehensive assessment at risk mental states
CAM	confusion assessment method
CARS-M	clinician administered rating scales for mania
CBC	complete blood count
CBT	cognitive behavioral therapy
CBZ	carbamazepine
CCK	cholecystokinin
CDT	carbohydrate deficient transferrin
CIWA	clinical institute withdrawal assessment
CIWA-Ar	clinical institute withdrawal assessment for alcohol revised
CJD	creutzfeldt-jakob disease
CK	creatine kinase
CLOZ	clozapine
CNS	central nervous system
CO	carbon monoxide
CONT	continuation
COPD	chronic obstructive pulmonary disease
CRF	corticotropin-releasing factor

CSF	cerebro spinal fluid		GI	gastro intestinal
CSTC	cortical-striatal-thalamo-cortical circuitry		GMC	general medical condition
			H1	histamine receptor
CT	computed tomography		HAM-D	hamilton depression rating scale
CXR	chest x-ray			
D2	dopamine d2 receptors		HDL	high-density lipoprotein
DA	dopamine		HIV	human immunodeficiency virus
DARF	drug accountability record form		IDS-C	inventory of depressive symptomatology - clinician rated
DIS	diagnostic interview schedule			
DSM	diagnostic and statistical manual of mental disorders		IM	intramuscular
			IPT	integrated physiological therapy
DSM-IV-TR	diagnostic and statistical manual of mental disorders fourth edition text revision		ISBD	international society for bi-polar disorders
			ISS	internal state scale
DSR	delirium rating scales		LDL	low density lipoprotien
ECG	electrocardiogram		LFT	liver function test
ECT	electroconvulsive therapy		Li	lithium
EEG	electroencephalogram		LP	lumbar puncture
eg	exempli gratia (for example)		LSD	lysergic acid diethylamide
EMDR	eye movement desensitization and reprocessing		MADRS	montgomery-asperg depression rating scale
EPS	extrapyramidal symptoms		MAOIs	monoamine oxidase inhibitors
ESR	erythrocyte sedimentation rate		MCMI-III	million clinical multiaxial inventory-iii
ETOH	ethyl alcohol (ethanol)			
FGA	first generation antipsychotics		MCV	mean corpuscular volume
GABA	gamma-amino butyric acid		MDAS	memorial delirium assessment scale
GAD	generalized anxiety disorder			
GAF	global assessment of functioning		MDE	major depressive episode
			MDMA	methylenedioxymethamphetamine
GGT	glutamyltransferase			
GHB	gamma-hydroxybutyric acid		MDD	major depressive disorder

MDQ	mood disorders questionnaire	PO4	phosphorus
MMPI-II	minnesota multiphasic personality inventory-ii	QTP	quetiapine
		RIS	risperidone
MMSE	mini-mental state examination	SADS	schedule for affective disorders and schizophrenia
MRI	magnetic resonance imaging	SCID	the structured clinical interview for the dsm-iv
NA	noradrenalin		
NASA	norepinephrine antagonist and serotonin antagonists	SGA	second generation antipsychotics
NE	norepinephrine	SL	sub lingual
NDRI	norepinephrine dopamine reuptake inhibitors	SNRIs	seratonin-norepinephrine reuptake inhibitors
NMDA	n -methyl- d -aspartate	SOPS	scale of prodromal symptoms
NMS	neuroleptic malignant syndrome	SPECT	single-photon emission computed tomography
NOS	not otherwise specified	SIPS	structured interview for prodromal symptoms
NPH	normal pressure hydrocephalus		
OCD	obsessive-compulsive disorder	SSRIs	selective serotonin reuptake inhibitors
OCPD	obsessive compulsive personality disorder	TAP	typical antipsychotic
		TCAs	tricyclic antidepressants
OD	once a day	TD	tardive dyskinesia
OLZ	olanzapine	TFT	thyroid function test
OXC	oxcarbazepine	TSH	thyroid stimulating harmone
PAS	premorbid assessment scale	US	united states
PCP	phencyclidine	VPA	valproate/valproic acid;
PD	personality disorder/dysfunction	WBC	white blood cells
PDD	pervasive developmental disorders	Y-BOCS	yale-brown obsessive compulsive scale
PDI	personality diagnostic inventory	YMRS	young mania rating scale
PET	positron emission tomography	yrs	years
PO	per os	ZIP	ziprasidone
PTSD	post traumatic stress disorder		

13.2 Useful Links/Websites

American Psychiatric Association
http://www.psych.org/

World Psychiatric Association
www.wpanet.org/

California Psychiatric Association
www.calpsych.org/

European Psychiatric Association
www.europsy.net/

Royal College of Psychiatrists
www.rcpsych.ac.uk/

American Psychoanalytic Association
http://www.apsa.org/

Canadian Psychiatric Association
www.cpa-apc.org/index.php

National Guideline Clearinghouse
http://www.guidelines.gov/content.aspx?id=9316

American Academy of Family Physicians ICD-9 Coding Tools
http://www.aafp.org/online/en/home/publications/journals/fpm/icd9.html

American Psychological Association
http://www.apa.org/

World Health Organization
The Alcohol Use Disorders Identification Test
http://whqlibdoc.who.int/hq/2001/WHO_MSD_MSB_01.6a.pdf

Michigan Implementation of Medication Algorithms (MIMA)
http://www.mirecovery.org/Portals/0/Pages/Recovery101/
MMA_Schizophrenia_081911.pdf

Trade name = **bold**   Drug name = *italic*

Trade name = **bold**   Drug name = *italic*

Trade name = **bold**   Drug name = *italic*

Trade name = **bold**   Drug name = *italic*

Trade name = bold   Drug name = italic

Trade name = **bold**   Drug name = *italic*

A Concise Clinical Reference Tool For Medical Interns and Residents

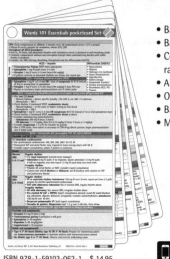

- Basic components of the history
- Basic outlines of ACLS algorithms
- Common lab values and normal ranges, important equations, etc.
- ABG interpretation
- Outlines of common notes
- Basic information on common drugs
- Must-knows and clinical pearls

ISBN 978-1-59103-062-1 $ 14.95

Available on the App Store

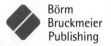

Börm
Bruckmeier
Publishing

A Concise Clinical Reference Tool For Medical Interns and Residents

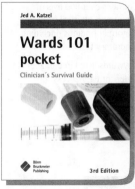

ISBN 978-1-59103-266-3 $ 19.95

- Basics such as important scales and scores, H&P, writing notes and orders
- The latest management and therapeutic recommendations for conditions in over 15 specialities
- More than 200 figures and tables for quick access to important information
- Includes neurology, ID, psychiatry, geriatrics, pediatrics and much more
- Extra information: normal values, medical formulas, common abbreviations, statistics

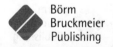

Börm
Bruckmeier
Publishing

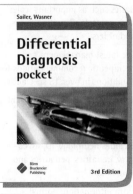

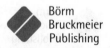

For Students, Nurses, and All Other Health Care Professionals

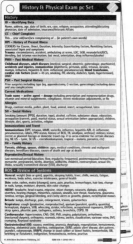

The new and extended History & Physical Examination pocketcard Set represents a vital resource for recognizing signs and symptoms and diagnosing. This efficiently arranged reference card offers:

- History and physical examination with notes on ID, CC, HPI, PMH, allergies, current medications, SH, FH, and sexual history

- In addition: GA, VS, MS, skin, lymph nodes, HEENT, neck, thorax, lungs, female breasts, CVS, abdomen, genitalia, rectum, musculoskeletal, neurologic system, and more

- Now with graphics for lung and heart auscultation and reflexes

ISBN 978-1-59103-097-3 $ 7.95

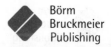

Börm Bruckmeier Publishing

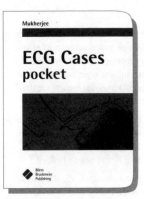

ISBN 978-1-59103-229-6
$ 16.95

- ECG Cases pocket provides 60 examples of common clinical problems encountered in the wards, emergency room, or outpatient sitting

- Each ECG is preceded by a brief clinical history and pertinent physical examination findings, so that the the tracings may be interpreted in the appropriate clinical context

- Detailed answers concentrate on the clinical interpretation of the clinical interpretation of the results and give advice on what to do

- The convinient size of this book will enable medical students, interns, residents, and other trainees to carry it in their pockets, for use as a quick reference

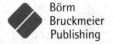

Börm
Bruckmeier
Publishing